Andropause: The Complete Male Menopause Guide

The Shocking Truth about Low Testosterone

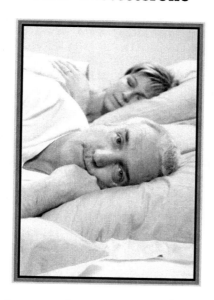

Discover the signs and symptoms of Low T, including proven treatments to combat the Andropause for a happier, healthier and more sexually-satisfying life.

Written By Brady Howard

DEDICATION

For my dad

Willie (Kay) Howard
1939 – 2012

Who instilled in me, an appreciation
for the joy of life.

ACKNOWLEDGMENTS

I'd like to express my gratitude to my beloved mother Lea for her ever-lasting encouragement for me to always dream big; and a very special thanks to my loving wife Nikki, who has loved and supported me for many years and stuck with me through seemingly endless hours of writing this important book.

To my wonderful children – you all are bar none the best kids any father could ever hope for and have brought a tremendous amount of joy and happiness into my life.

Thanks to all my friends and family, but particularly Wayne whose sage advice and dedicated friendship over the years helped to inspire me. I'd like to also thank Michael (my brother from the mile high city) for his key insights shared about the medical industry amongst countless other topics; and to my buddy Dr. Jay and his team of researchers for their valuable contributions towards this extraordinary book project.

To All of You,
a Big Huge
Thank You...

CONTENTS

CHAPTER 1 WHAT IS ANDROPAUSE? 1

CHAPTER 2 ANDROPAUSE IN HISTORY 13

CHAPTER 3 SOME FACTS ABOUT ANDROPAUSE 24

CHAPTER 4 THE IMPACT OF ANDROPAUSE ON THE BODY AND MIND 30

CHAPTER 5 HOW TESTOSTERONE WORKS 39

CHAPTER 6 DIAGNOSING ANDROPAUSE 46

CHAPTER 7 GMOS – GENETIC MODIFICATION OF OUR FOODS . 60

CHAPTER 8 THE PROSTATE AND IMPOTENCE 69

CHAPTER 9 DIET, EXERCISE AND ANDROPAUSE 82

CHAPTER 10 LIVING WITH ANDROPAUSE & TREATMENT 98

CHAPTER 11 ALTERNATIVE TREATMENT METHODS 105

BIBLIOGRAPHY 126

FOLLOW THE PLAN 127

INDEX 128

This Page Is Intentionally Blank

CHAPTER 1

WHAT IS ANDROPAUSE?

Definition (Wikipedia):
Andropause which is a term assigned to **male menopause**, also sometimes referred to as "mano-pause", has earned this nickname in some parts of the world, because of a set of symptoms or effects that takes place in the majority of men who are aging, and these have some similarities to the menopause effects that women have.

Andropause may be related to the slow but steady reduction in production of the hormones Testosterone and Dehydro-epiandrosterone in middle-aged men, and the symptoms and consequences that appear as a result of that reduction.

That reduction is also linked to a reduction in <u>Leydig cells,</u> (also called the interstitial cells of Leydig, which are located right next to the testicles seminiferous tubules. The Leydig cells are responsible for the production of Testosterone which the luteinizing hormone (LH) is present. A gradual declination in the level of Testosterone occurs with age, in both men and women, and this has been extremely well recorded.

Hard as it is for some men to believe, the term "Andropause" is not presently recognized by the <u>World Health Organization</u> while "menopause" which has similar symptoms is indeed recognized. Understandably, the words are oftentimes used interchangeably by many people, and can at times be confusing as well.

In the following pages, we will delve deeply into what this condition looks like, how it impacts the body, and how its effects can be mitigated to provide a better quality of life for you.

After all, that is why you are reading this book, isn't it? If you are looking for really honest information about male menopause, this book will certainly help you better understand the changes you may be currently experiencing, along with bona-fide solutions that have been proven to work for many men around the world.

This newfound understanding will help to remove any fear, as you discover the little known options available for you to successfully transform this phase of your life into just another natural process that can be easily managed.

As Heraclitus once said, "The only thing constant is change"…. and change is nothing to fear.

> ### Remember when you were young and you couldn't wait to grow up; what the hell were you thinking?

Are you feeling tired or run down?

For many men, this may sound all too familiar. Perhaps your libido isn't what it once was or it seems harder than ever to stay-in-shape. Most people know that women experience menopause and it is certainly the butt of many jokes, (like maybe it should be called 'womenopause') but were you even aware that men experience a parallel type of male menopause as well?

For men who believe they are going through the proverbial "mid-life crisis", some doctors and researchers say you may actually be experiencing a form of "male menopause" or, more accurately, "Andropause."

Andropause is a male phenomenon similar to the female menopause that happens to a lot of us later in life.

Often jokingly referred to as 'mano-pause' in general conversation, it's hardly a laughing matter, especially for most men currently going through it.

MIDDLE AGE IS THE STARTING LINE

It is hard to predict at what exact age the symptoms will begin to kick-in-full for any given person. That's simply because every man may experience different symptoms. However, evidence seems to suggest that Andropause affects most middle-aged men between forty to fifty (40-50) years old. However, unlike female menopause, Andropause has no obvious or visible external markers to show its presence, and it tends to take place over an extended period of time, gradually... and never all at once.

This subtlety can make it feel very unnerving and mysterious, creating fear and apprehension because you may not notice exactly why you are feeling the way you do. All you know is that you've changed somehow and how can you "fix it" if you can't quite exactly put your finger on the cause? Due to various contributing factors, Andropause may be a difficult thing to live with. It can be hard on you, your spouse, your family, your friends, and even your co-workers as it impacts just about everyone around you.

Unlike female menopause, the gradual transition that men go through with Andropause can span as long as 20 to 30 years or more. During this span of time we may notice the quality of our attitude decline. This seems to be perfectly natural considering that not so long ago, we were young and virile. The world was our oyster and we felt powerful and vital. Our attitude can sour when we suddenly realize that we can't do the things we used to do but we don't know why. It's not something obvious and we can't quite recall exactly when it started.

This uncertainty can then easily manifest into growing psychological stresses. One day, our partner does or says something rather innocent or benign that triggers an uncharacteristic outburst of anger. It never used to bother us before and now we feel surprised and confused by our over-reaction. "What was I thinking? Why did that upset me so much? What is wrong with me?" As the stress builds, it is not unusual for many men to ramp up habitual behaviors to cope with the anxiety.

The downward spiral could then lead to increased smoking, alcohol and/or drug use. Maybe you were a 'social drinker' before but your use quickly becomes abuse to mask the fear building within that you are somehow losing control over your life. The abuse of these common escape mechanisms, to numb the anxiety and uncertainty, including prescription medications, is often a recipe for disaster. You're a smart guy, you can read labels and you know better than to drink and drive. Sure, you do but you are in pain, suffering mental anguish and then the injuries start to happen.

You may be suffering more injuries than usual, due to your diminished reflexes from alcohol, drugs or simply a reduction in muscle strength and flexibility because, hey, you're no spring chicken anymore! Now you may find yourself with broken limbs or even more serious injuries requiring surgery (and, of course, plenty of prescription drugs and pain medications to go along with it). For a man to admit he's not strong is a very difficult thing and nothing will knock you down quicker than a debilitating surgery that leaves you feeling helpless or bed-ridden for extended periods of time.

As you can imagine, and maybe you've actually been through it yourself, this condition could lead straight into depression and obesity. Or vice versa. Either way, you've been sidelined and you're perhaps physically unable to exercise. This is a tough hole to climb out of and extended illnesses and recovery from major surgeries provide a slippery slope of depression and risk of further complications when your immune system isn't working as effectively as it should and you're feeling 'down and out.'

Perhaps there's a defiant voice inside you that's saying, "But that's just the hard knocks of life. Everybody goes through that at one time or another and it doesn't mean they have Andropause." You're right. These things do happen and you might come through it just fine. It's also very important to make sure you are honest with yourself and rule out Andropause because if you have it, it is treatable and manageable. The first step is a proper diagnosis.

CAUSES AND EFFECTS OF ANDROPAUSE

So, what causes it you might ask? From a purely scientific standpoint, Andropause is defined simply as a drop in male hormones. Really, it is so much more than that. This decline in male hormones triggers a complex mix of symptoms in middle-aged men. Gradually, over time, you may start to notice physical changes in your body, changes in attitude, motivation, energy levels and/or even libido.

You might experience weight gain or erectile dysfunction, depression, loss of energy and sex drive or even physical endurance. The lowering of Testosterone can also bring about the threat of other health risks for men, such as heart disease, osteoporosis, insulin resistance, and even Alzheimer's disease.

Unfortunately, because of considerable skepticism, even in this modern day and age, it's still difficult to find treatment for this condition, beyond the standard response of "you're just getting older". The World Health Organization does not even recognize the term "Andropause", even while it does give female "menopause" credibility as a very real and serious medical condition.

Unless you have an extremely progressive physician, more often than not you'll be told to simply "shake it off and buck up."

You need to be armed with some facts, straight talk and professional support to tackle this condition so let's talk about what we do know…

1. **Testosterone is of major importance to the male body:** It is manufactured by your testicles (testes) and also, is a function of your adrenal glands. It is of key importance to the man as the hormone Estrogen is to a woman.

   Testosterone is mandatory for normal sexual function and is responsible for enabling erections. It also helps the male to buildup essential proteins within the body.

2. **Testosterone decline is normal:** Though a natural decline in Testosterone levels is a given for virtually all men as they age, there is absolutely no way to predict who will end up with the actual condition called Andropause, which necessitates treatment to overcome.

3. **Testosterone levels impact your body:** Testosterone levels have a major influence on multiple metabolic activities within your body, including producing healthy blood cells though your bone marrow, the production and structuring of healthy bone, healthy function of the liver, growth of the prostate gland, as well as metabolizing of fat and carbohydrates.

   Testosterone also impacts libido, your mood, hair growth or loss (balding), sebum production, the strength and density of muscles. Testosterone also modulates the body's immune system to help combat illness and disease.

4. **Andropause is not a new phenomenon:** The first description of this condition in medical literature can be found as early as the 1940's. In 1944, two physicians

began diagnosing symptoms that they called male climacteric, which had symptoms of decreased sex drive, loss of memory, depression, extreme fatigue levels, and unstable sleep patterns. Their discovery was based on all these symptoms being linked to low Testosterone levels in their patient's blood. But, even as old as the phenomenon is, the ability to accurately diagnose it is still little understood and involves using fairly new technology.

5. **Testing is available:** The highly sensitive test required for determining bio-available Testosterone was not available until recently, meaning that men suffering from this condition not very long ago suffered for a long time because their Andropause was either underdiagnosed or undertreated. Fortunately, there's a lot of exciting research on the horizon aimed at developing new, more advanced testing methods.

MEDICAL RESEARCH ON ANDROPAUSE

According to the Cleveland Clinic of Ohio, the world's leading clinic on treating many forms of sexual dysfunction, there's heated debate among some health care professionals about whether or not men really do go through a well-defined form of menopause.

While researchers at Northwestern Memorial Hospital in Chicago, estimate that approximately five million men in the United States are affected by Andropause, treatment is not readily available or provided at a sufficient level to even come close to addressing that many patients. And it would help if they could start by agreeing on the terminology they use to talk about it.

ANDROPAUSE VS HYPOGONADISM

Some of those in the medical field who do believe in the existence of the Andropause phenomenon do not refer to it as male menopause; what we've been referring to as Andropause.

Instead, they will use terms such as Testosterone deficiency or late-onset Hypogonadism.

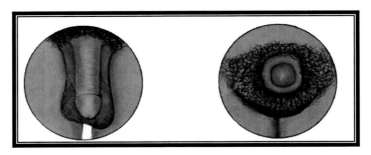

This is an image of normal function to extreme Hypogonadism

Hypogonadism refers to Testosterone levels that are considered too low for the naturally occurring decline in Testosterone experienced by an aging man.

Late-onset Hypogonadism can be put alongside the common place understanding of male menopause and their symptoms are very comparable and similar, even though they are two separate conditions. To further clarify this difference, Hypogonadism specifically refers to the occurrence where the testicles no longer produce enough Testosterone.

As you may well know, Testosterone is the key hormone in masculine growth and development. It is essentially what makes a man a man. When this drop in Testosterone level occurs, men go through significant physical and mental changes that can mirror Andropause. So, in that regard, Hypogonadism could be said to be one symptom of Andropause. Likewise, having one, does not necessitate the other.

EMERGING SCIENTIFIC DATA
Men are living much longer thanks to many advances in the medical field and therefore, there has also been a rapidly-growing interest in Andropause. Naturally, this increased interest will spur

more research to develop new methods to effectively diagnose, treat and manage it.

In Canada, Andropause has gained a lot of attention in recent years which has resulted in a massive effort by some American-based medical researchers to quickly share the latest emerging scientific data with Canadian physicians.

SHBG AND BIO-AVAILABLE TESTOSTERONE

Starting at somewhere around forty (40) years of age, the aging man's Testosterone levels begin dropping by about 10% every decade. Right around the time this begins to happen, something else known as Sex Hormone-Binding Globulin (or SHBG), steadily rises.

As the SHBG increases, it traps the majority of the body's available circulating Testosterone and makes it unavailable to be used by the body's tissues for all the important functions we've mentioned before. The 'free' Testosterone that remains in circulation tries to carry on the best it can to do all the beneficial work it's responsible for. In a nutshell, you have less and less Testosterone trying to do the same amount of work it's always been required to do in an effort to ensure a healthy body.

This remaining Testosterone is called 'bio-available' Testosterone and will decline for every man, the older they get. Some men will drop to lower levels than others. When this 'Bio-available' Testosterone is found to be at lower than normal levels, as previously described by the term Hypogonadism, medical doctors will oftentimes associate this with Andropause.

SYMPTOMOLOGY IMPACTS THE QUALITY OF LIFE

Symptoms following the drop in Testosterone impact the quality of a man's life. It seems that now, approximately 30% of the male population who have reached their 50th birthday are experiencing lowered Testosterone in the blood streams, low enough to result in Andropause symptomology. When the male body has less bio-available Testosterone, it can bring about radical changes.

ORGANIC FAILURE BEGINS
These radical changes target organs that need Testosterone to function properly, and thus organs no longer do so. This is a warning that the body needs help, and fast.

CHANGES ARE DIFFERENT FROM MAN TO MAN
Not all men experience the same changes to the same extent, this is related to the variation in Testosterone levels in healthy men.

The typical male body responds to having this low level of bio-available Testosterone with a diminished desire for sex, as well as considerable changes within your emotional base, psychological stability and last but not least, oftentimes you will experience unwelcomed behavioral changes. There is also decreased muscle mass, loss of muscle strength, and increased upper and central body fat.

SILENT AND DEADLY
While Andropause's impact on a man's quality of life is drastic, it does have other long-term effects that are silent and harder to track. The two that are most notable are the increase in cardiovascular risks and osteoporosis. The bone tissue of a healthy person is another reason Andropause has gone underdiagnosed over the years, due to the vagueness of symptoms and the realization that symptomology can vary greatly among individuals who are impacted by this life-changing condition.

ACCEPTING THE PROBLEM IS DIFFICULT
In many cases, some men can't honestly admit to themselves that they've got a problem, down there, with the functioning of their sex lives and energy levels. Psychologically, however, the impact for a formerly sexually active man can be quite devastating.

Added to that, physicians haven't always considered low Testosterone levels a possible cause stemming from other underlying health issues.

Doctors in the recent past have often mistakenly concluded that Andropause symptomology is only associated with some other health condition such as being depressed, or it was simply caused by the normal process of aging.

This type of lax attitude by a medical doctor has led them to simply brush off the symptoms by telling their patients to just accept the inevitable.

OSTEOPOROSIS ISN'T JUST A WOMEN'S DISEASE
We've heard for years about many women after having endured menopause, then being subject to suffering from osteoporosis or weakened bones. This is mainly related to their drop in Estrogen.

In men, aged from 40 to 70 years, the density of their bone tissue declines up to 15% due to Testosterone depletion.

Testosterone's role in our health includes helping maintain healthy bones. Lower Testosterone levels equals lower bone density in the long run... which could result in osteoporosis.

OSTEOPOROSIS IN MEN
Twelve (12) percent of men over the age of 50, have developed osteoporosis. (www.wikipedia.com) Hip fractures reported to physicians and hospitals are on the rise in aging men as it is in females of the same age group. These are particularly devastating because one third (1/3) of male patients with osteoporosis never seem to regain full mobility.

OSTEOPOROSIS INCREASING IN CANADA
Canada reports that 20-30% of the osteoporotic fractures in the elderly are now occurring in older men, and it seems that figure is on the rise. Cases of women with osteoporosis fractures is already

stabilizing, no doubt due to improvement of lifestyle, adding calcium supplements and from taking advantage of hormone replacement therapies.

SOMETHING FOR MEN TO WORRY ABOUT

A few reasons osteoporosis in men, due to lower bone density, is something to worry about includes: men discover that they are at risk due to lowered bone density – at risk for frequent falls, fractures, and the miserable pain that comes along with it. And, all too often, with many fall cases, there's a loss of independence.

The most common areas that are affected by osteoporosis are the wrists, hips, spine and ribs.

GOT ROUNDED SHOULDERS?

Another slow but progressive consequence of osteoporosis is rounding of the shoulders and the gradual loss of height over time.

HEART RISKS ALSO

One must also take note of the cardiovascular risk, it is now widely accepted that after menopause a woman's risk of hardened arteries, known as atherosclerosis, may increase. Women's Hormone Replacement Therapy (Estrogen), overall, tends to eliminate this problem.

New studies indicate that something similar occurs in men when they age and their T-levels drop. Thus far, the research for men isn't as nearly complete as that of women, and additional funding will help with this, but already the findings of clinical trials demonstrate that there is an absolute correlation between male low T-levels and a rise in cardiovascular health issues in men.

CHAPTER 2

ANDROPAUSE IN HISTORY

By the nineteenth and early twentieth century, writers everywhere were talking about "the change" for men and women alike. While most of this writing worked to dispel the commonplace aura of anxiety surrounding the popular topic and to encourage middle-aged women (and their husbands) to take this change gracefully, there wasn't a lot of information out there beyond the fact that it would happen to each and every one of us eventually.

Overtime, regardless of what was or was not known about it, menopause was generally accepted as a necessary yet transitory phase through which the majority of those impacted would pass on to a higher and more refined stage of life.

MALE MENOPAUSE BUZZES THE WORLD

During the 1930's, male menopause became quite the buzz, appearing in everything from TIME magazine articles to the local news channel and that terminology continued to be popular through the 1950's until it practically vanished, never to be heard from again. Or so we thought...

It was miraculously picked up as a trendy topic in the early 1990's and writing on the subject began again.

EARLY RESEARCH AND 'MANOPAUSE'

It was in 1944, when medical researchers Carl Heller and Gordon Myers acknowledged their discovery of indications of what they would refer to as the "male climacteric," (climacteric is an alternative expression for menopause). Their description of climacteric included the loss of sex urge, forms of depression, difficulty focusing, sweats and hot flashes.

Similarly, a colloquial expression "man-o-pause" was later named as an obvious homage to the feminine affliction, to help explain all of the physical, emotional and mental changes that so many men begin to experience, starting in their middle years.

Others called it a "mid-life crisis," leading popular media to link "mano-pause" to an image of 50-something male with greying hair purchasing a quarter million dollar Lamborghini (or something closer to his price range), then quitting his job and going out on his own or changing the job he's had for something completely different, or... the big game changer - hooking up with women half his age!

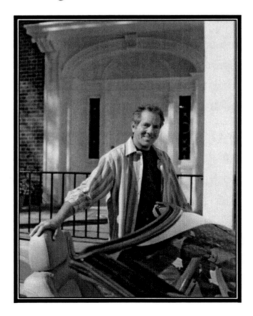

This signals a time in a man's life when he seems most compelled to turn everything upside down in rebellion against a loss of youth, vigor and all the trappings associated with his masculinity.

Over the years, scientific opinions have ranged anywhere from calling the Andropause - male menopause phenomenon - "debatable at best" to citing it as one of the most common causes of depression in the older male. Whether or not the medical world believes in it does not deter, however, the physical impact that having a reduced Testosterone level has on the average man is very much real indeed.

THE MID-LIFE CRISIS VS ANDROPAUSE

The first notion of something like a mid-life crisis began with followers of the legendary Austrian neurologist, Sigmund Freud, commonly referred to as the founding father of psychoanalysis.

He believed that everyone's thoughts during middle age were steered by their suppressed fear that half their life was over, and sooner or later, usually sooner, they would be dying. The psychological moniker 'Mid-life Crisis' was actually first coined by a Canadian psychoanalyst named Elliott Jaques in 1965, when he defined it as a time in an adult's life where they've come to realize the existence of their own mortality.

It goes something like this. When they hit a certain age, men begin thinking about their past accomplishments and current situation and suddenly come to realize that their life is nearly half over. Then it feels like the clock is quickly ticking away and there isn't enough time to do those things you haven't yet done. This realization happens to many people during the mid-life transition.

In some instances, a crisis is brought on by a sudden transition occurring in the middle-age years, things such as the onset of Andropause, the death of one's parents/family or close friends, or any number of other significant or real tragic life events.

If you're unemployed or facing unemployment, or realize that you really and truly hate your job or career and you're really feeling stuck with no chance of escape, these thoughts and feelings can understandably make you reassess your dreams, goals or ambitions. This reassessment can also bring about sudden changes in a persons' day-to-day experience of life. Suddenly there is a change in their work life, in their work-to-life harmony, marriage or other committed relationship, and you may be compelled to make unusually large cash expenditures or undergo a dramatic change in your physical appearance.

Or, maybe you're just going through a phase?

However, the thought of a mid-life crisis being just a phase that the majority of adults go through was rejected in the 1980's by academic research. The result of one study showed that less than 10% of those in the U.S. ever felt a psychological crisis due to their age, or due to aging in general.

It's believed that individual personality and a history of psychological crisis predisposes some people for a 'traditional' mid-life crisis, while others make it through their whole lives without such an episode. However, those that go through it suffer from a variety of symptoms and show a wide range of behaviors that smack of desperation.

At this point in our discussion, I think it's important to make a clear distinction of what a 'mid-life crisis' is and what a mid-life stressor is.

MID-LIFE CRISIS OR MID-LIFE STRESSOR?
Mid-life is a period of time, often referred to as the years between 40 and 60, whereby one oftentimes finds him/herself reflecting upon all of the successes, failures and regrets experienced throughout their lives.

However, even with this knowledge, the majority of mid-life stressors are still incorrectly labeled as mid-life crises.

David Almeida, Professor – Dept. of Human Development and Family Studies at Penn State University, is a life-span developmental psychologist. He suggests that simple day-to-day stressors eventually just add up and become too much for us to bear. Thus people oftentimes inappropriately think of this as if it were a crisis. In reality, it's just an 'overload' of stress as a result of that persons' exceedingly overwhelmed life experience.

Things such as a career setback or the death of a loved one can cause stress or depression in normal middle-age adults. However, if these major life events took place earlier in life or at a later stage in your life, they still might be a crisis, but not related to the mid-life stage of life. In the same study mentioned earlier, 15% of middle-aged adults, had experienced similar forms of turmoil during their mid-life stage.

There have been other studies that suggest culture has something to do with mid-life crisis. Interestingly, one such study found that this phenomenon is almost absent in Japanese and Indian cultures. This startling fact suggests that a mid-life crisis could be merely a cultural construct. The authors of the study hypothesized that Western societies have popularized the mid-life crisis concept due to their pervasive "culture of youth."

Research has also found that reflection and reassessment are a natural part of middle-age, and do not always result in psychological upheaval characterized by a mid-life crisis.

MID-LIFE CRISIS STUDY

A larger study done in the 1990's discovered that 45 years old was the approximate age for men having the onset of a mid-life crisis.

Age-related mid-life crisis is most often apparent from 41 to 60 years of age in about 10% of the middle-aged adults who go through it. The length of these crises seems to differ based on gender; in women it lasts 2-5 years, while in men the time is much longer (3-10 years or more).

The existence, let alone the treatment of a mid-life crisis, like the treatment of Andropause, has been also been met with criticism by opponents. In the case of this phenomenon, another study found that 23% of the participants claimed they suffered from what they called a 'mid-life crisis'.

Upon further investigation the researchers discovered that only 8% of them stated their crisis was due to their realizations about aging, while the remaining 15% had indeed had significant life changes or experienced losses such as divorce or losing of a job. This makes a case for a multitude of mid-life stressors, as opposed to a mid-life crisis, per se.

OTHER POSSIBLE CAUSATIONS

Other possible causes for a mid-life crisis, outside of aging itself, are a combination of changes, problems and regrets in one's life.

In one way or another we have allotted ourselves only a specific amount of time to achieve specific life goals. We determine this based on our own ideals or those of influential people around us; our parents, for example.

- **Personal expectations:**
  We expect our jobs or careers to reach a certain level by a certain age, and if we're lacking a job at middle-age the crisis is worse. Another area that the majority of us put a time stamp on is marriage. Lack of a spousal relationship in mid-life is alarming to most of the older generations.

- **Empty nest syndrome:**
  When our children mature and leave home, and they have been in close proximity to us since birth, it can be a startling and life-changing experience.

  Also, the lack of having children, when a man or woman reaches a certain age, can have a unique impact, especially if there is environmental or social pressure to have a child.

- **A sense of lack:**
  While noticing things that are lacking in our lives at middle-age, the realization that our parents are aging, if they have not passed on already, once again awakens us to our own mortality.
- **The aging of our bodies:**
  The physical changes often associated with aging also wakes us up to the fact that we are indeed aging ourselves and have a limited amount of time to live in this world.

MEN AND WOMEN HANDLE IT DIFFERENTLY

Men and women seem to approach a mid-life crisis very differently. As was briefly noted before, the popular American stereotype of a man going through his change of life is often depicted by him going out to purchase an expensive sports car that he has no real need for or cannot afford. A woman, on the other hand, may grab a half gallon of ice cream and a spoon.

Research has also shown that the triggers are different by gender as well. Men are more likely to go into crisis over work issues because they traditionally define themselves by their careers and how much money they have in the bank. Women tend to focus on personal evaluations of their roles in life.

Though men and women arrive at their own personal state of mid-life crisis via different routes, the emotions they feel and the general malaise about the condition are very similar. The extreme emotions they experience and try to cope with in different ways range from general anxiety to extreme panic and every emotion in between.

PSYCHOLOGICAL FACTORS

Some psychologists believe that in the case of men, their experience of a crisis at mid-life is due to the psychological response to their spouses reaching menopause, the end of their reproductive lives. In my opinion this is pure hypothesis, as it says that men are more attracted to reproductive or fertile women in general than to their wives, specifically.

Having spoken to many men about this issue, I've concluded that while they may be attracted to younger women, by and large they are basically faithful men due to their character. They seem to reframe the experience and convince themselves that their wives have become their own personal classic sports model. Most of them believe they don't need any other woman.

A main assumption of a mid-life crisis is that being in the middle age group brings on drastic, and often negative, changes in a person's life. They assume their lives are either going to be filled with negative events or be extremely stressful to them. In addition, middle aged men can often feel as if they're watching the quality of their lives take a drastic nose-dive for the worse.

When experiencing Andropause or a mid-life crisis it's common to have some of the following feelings:

- The sudden search for an unrealized dream or goal you may have previously neglected or missed out on.

- A deep sense of remorse for goals you set that you have yet to act on or accomplish.

- A heightened awareness of more successful relatives or colleagues and the fear of feeling humiliated when with them.

- A wanting, more than anything, to regain your feelings of youthfulness despite your age.

- The urge to spend more time by oneself, or only with specific friends.

It is also common to exhibit some of the following behaviors in response to a mid-life crisis or awareness of Andropause:

- Abusing alcohol, drugs or an addiction to pornography.

- Obsession in acquiring costly material things such as an exotic motorcycle, boat, sports car, or expensive decorative jewelry including watches, rings, bracelets, or necklaces. Discovering a new sense of depression.

- Feeling overwhelming remorse for wrongs you may have done throughout your life and a desire to "make right".

- Beginning to pay special attention to your physical appearance. Covering baldness, changing hair color, hiding signs of aging, or wearing trendy clothing styled for much younger persons (i.e., skinny jeans), and/or a crazed interest to deface their bodies with tattoos or piercings, or engage in other practices they would not normally do otherwise.

- Hanging around with much younger people and getting into relationships with them. (Friendships, mentor relationships, sexual relationships, inappropriate professional situations, etc.)

- And sometimes putting unwarranted pressure (at a level which psychologists and educators feel is damaging) on your children to be the absolute best in academics, sports, and/or the creative arts - but never in that order.

MID-LIFE CRISIS PREVENTION AND TREATMENT

Regardless of how you feel about it, or your beliefs about its causes and effects - there are things you can do to better manage and even prevent a crisis from happening to you.

The logical choice is to make certain fundamental changes earlier on in your life to help you prevent a 'mid-life' crisis, and Andropause. These would include changing your job or career path sooner, rather than waiting for some more opportune time in the future. Take the proverbial "bull by the horns" now, while you are more easily able to handle such a large transition.

If you are considering going back to school or changing your major, it's better to do this sooner rather than later, to give yourself time to adjust to a new learning curve. In essence, get on with those and any other things you want to do that you keep putting off for tomorrow. Procrastination is the straightest path to regret that can haunt you later in life. But what if you are already in mid-life?

Think of this time in your life as a transitional phase. Psychologists often recommend that Andropause, Mid-life Crisis and Erectile Dysfunction be treated as a transitional phase of life, very much like the rebellious teenage years that lead up to adulthood. In the case of Mid-Life Crisis and Andropause they suggest that it is the period of a rebellious adult leading up to old age, and that there's no need to go down fighting.

This concept helps us to view this life changing experience as an opportunity for new experiences, positive personal growth and a chance to mentally prepare oneself for aging. This sort of mental preparation can often effect a reduction in those overwhelming emotional feelings that often lead to the crisis stage.

BASK IN YOUR OWN GLORY INSTEAD

For most men, after 40 is a time to bask with great satisfaction in their life accomplishments, however, the passage into middle-age isn't the same for everyone. While the symptoms of depression, change in mood, and behavior are found in mid-life crisis, Andropause is far more complex on a deeper level.

It has more to do with hormones and the way the body itself functions with lower levels of hormones.

HERBAL THERAPIES

The Traditional Chinese, astrologers and physicians alike, studied everything, from the stars to the planets and everything in between just to learn how to bring harmony to the human body in a more natural way.

They understood that all must be in place for a clean system, including the hormonal balance of both men and women. Herbs such as Tribulus Terrestris (bai-ji-li, in the field of Traditional Chinese Herbology) were given to aging men to help combat "The Change".

Tribulus Terrestris was also used as a constituent tonic in Indian Ayurveda practice, where it is known to help increase natural masculine hormones.

According to Examine.com, the roots of the Tribulus Terrestri can enhance the male sex drive and improves human sexual well-being without affecting Testosterone and the fruit itself demonstrates to be powerfully defensive of organ operation.

Furthermore, the herb also appears to have cardiovascular benefits as well. Fortunately today, Andropause is becoming more widely accepted as a normal, treatable occurrence and Herbal therapies are at the forefront of treatment options.

Next we'll delve deeper into the details of the physiology of Andropause and its effects.

CHAPTER 3

SOME FACTS ABOUT ANDROPAUSE

Because of the resistance of the medical field to assign a diagnostic code for Andropause, there is no worldwide statistic available. With the World Health Organization refusing to recognize or support the diagnosis at the time of this writing, it's difficult to capture some much needed data to solidify its legitimacy and improve diagnosis and treatment.

From what we know, there are probably more than the estimated 25,000,000 males suffering from Andropause right now in the United States alone. And, that accounts for more than fifteen percent (15%) of the country's estimated male population.

HORMONAL NORMALCY IS CRITICAL

Complex hormonal cycles that impact moods, the well-being of our physical body, and the well-being of our sexual selves, impacts both men and women when they go through the reduced hormone production that typically occurs during mid-life.

The emotional symptoms of Andropause may include:

- Apprehension, anxiety, fear,

- Bad temper, bad/irritable mood,

- Melancholy, despair, hopelessness, and,

- Personal indeterminacy.

These emotional symptoms tend to mimic those experienced by women in menopause.

But there are more physical symptoms in men that are highly disturbing and cause long-term problems. Here are a few of the physical symptomology of the male menopause:

- Low energy, exhaustion, being weary, weakness,
- Loss of short-term memory and recall,
- Excessive weight gain, and
- Suffering from sleep disorders (i.e., sleep apnea).

Then we have the highly reviled sexual symptomology of Andropause:

- Reduced sex drive
- Erectile Dysfunction
- And, the common fear of inability to perform sexually.

Obviously, many guys always want to prove to others that he still is a sexual athlete.

As a result, Andropausal men may tend to search for a younger sex partner thinking that being with a younger person will provide some of the needed additional psychological stimulation to help fill the penile tissues with blood to produce a firmer erection. They mistakenly believe that it will help with their hormonal issues, which have nothing to do with the matter at all.

What will really alarm you is this statistic: a startling 52% of males from the ages of 40 to 70 already are now suffering, to some degree, from some manner of ED that is directly related to them having problems of Andropause.

Men who are experiencing the symptomology of Andropause tend to question and then evaluate their own identity, to wonder about the future with their own sexuality, dependence on others as they get older, and independence, whether they will be able to have it or not.

It's a lot like going through puberty all over again, and I'm sure you can recall how much fun that was! Many of these issues are directly related to and impacted by your Testosterone levels, or T-levels, for short. In puberty, you experienced this hormone kicking in to overdrive and there's bound to be some turbulence once the levels you were accustomed to as a young adult begin to subside/decrease.

WHAT YOUR T-LEVEL SHOULD BE

According to the Mayo Clinic, a healthy adult male Testosterone level should be 300 to 1,200 ng/dL (nanograms per deciliter). As you may have guessed, the male level of Testosterone normally peaks when he is in his 20's.

Starting just after 30 years of age, the average male T-Level begins to decline by 1% annually. Fifty years later, he's 80, and his T-level has dropped below 50% of the pre-Andropause level. His tank is less than half full, and that can certainly have a severe impact on him.

Let's discuss what's in store for your future unless you address your T-Levels, and I'll be straightforward in saying this …

THE LOWER YOUR T-LEVEL – THE FASTER YOU DIE

Validity of research indicates that men having lower than normal T-levels, had a much higher mortality rate than men with T-levels that were in the normal range. And, sadly – medical research has discovered that many of the sufferers have no clue that they even have lower Testosterone levels unless their doctor runs tests to diagnose specifically for Testosterone levels.

It's rare that the test is even ordered during a normal annual physical unless specifically requested by the patient.

LET'S TALK TESTOSTERONE THERAPY

However, before we do that, let me add that up to 25% of men 30 years old and older have already begun to experience the beginning of lower T-levels, and less than 5% of those men demonstrate symptomology sufficient to warrant testing and Testosterone therapy.

The more physicians become aware of and support the existence of Andropause, the more the available Testosterone gels, shots and patches will be prescribed as the first-line of treatment for most men experiencing a significant drop in their T-Levels.

One encouraging statistic cites the number of prescriptions filled in the United States between 1999 and 2008. The use of these forms of treatment increased by more than four-fold, to 3.3 million in 9 years.

Even with symptoms being rare, some physicians have started testing their middle-aged male patients for low Testosterone levels. Unfortunately, there is still some confusion when it comes to correctly diagnosing the symptoms of that 5% that clearly display them. This is due to the evidence of those same symptoms in cases that do not test low in Testosterone. They can be the result of other health problems including depression, stress or even heart disease.

BREAKTHROUGHS IN SYMPTOM RESEARCH

For the first time, in the early part of 2010, a group of researchers in Great Britain tried to isolate which symptoms were linked closest to low Testosterone levels. What they discovered was quite amazing and had far reaching implications for the accurate diagnosis of Andropause sufferers.

Their findings have shown there are only three reliable symptoms out of the multitude experienced that clearly point to low T-levels related to this affliction:

- Inability to have normal erections,

- Morning erections are few and far between,
- Thoughts of a sexual nature are disappearing.

The researchers also identified three other symptoms that were not linked to low Testosterone at all. These include:

- Low energy,
- Fatigue,
- Trouble engaging in physical activities.

The study concluded that there were fewer men suffering from male menopause than was previously thought; that only 2% of those were from 40 and 80.

These findings, and other research as well, also suggest that unless low Testosterone levels and menopause-like symptoms occur simultaneously, treatment is uncalled for.

Their reasoning relates to the risks of serious side effects in treating men who are of middle-age or older with Testosterone treatments. These side effects include:

- Coronary artery disease,
- Fluid retention,
- Alteration of serum lipid profile,
- Liver toxicity,
- Polycythemia,
- Prostate disease,
- Sleep apnea and,
- Impairment of spermatogenesis.

Although this research seems to indicate that Andropause is fairly uncommon, there is a reality that men must face.

The chances of developing it increase significantly as we age, as is shown in the chart below.

AGES	PERCENTAGE OF MEN AFFECTED
40 – 49	2% - 5%
50 – 59	6% - 40%
60 – 69	20% - 45%
70 – 79	34% - 70%
80 and older	91%

While the treatment is a complete science, the statistics are not. This does not mean however that symptoms should be ignored at any age. It's best to err on the side of caution, so do not hesitate to check with your doctor to be sure.

Here are some more interesting statistics to consider.

There are approximately 4 to 5 million men who currently have low Testosterone levels. Sadly, only 5 to 10 percent of these suffering millions of men will ever seek medical treatment for their condition.

A recent report by the World Health Organization has indicated that Testosterone levels in 70 year old men was only 10% of that found in 25 year olds.

That's a lot less than noted earlier and a frightening statistic to think about as we reach our golden years. This is especially true when you understand exactly how these low T-levels impact other bodily functions.

CHAPTER 4

THE IMPACT OF ANDROPAUSE ON THE

BODY AND MIND

Sex is really a remarkably complex process in human beings and it serves not only a biological purpose, but also psychological and social functions as well.

That being said, of all the many different organs, glands and entire systems in the body which are responsible for coordinating sexual response, the brain actually plays the central role in sexual functions. Surprised?

There are multiple structures in the brain that are practically time-locked to activate only during sexual arousal.

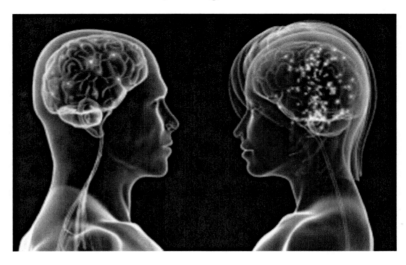

BRAIN INVOLVEMENT
In males the frontal and temporal lobes, cingulate cortex and subcortical areas of the brain have been shown to respond in direct association with sexual activity and arousal.

For example, the frontal lobe of the brain is responsible for the ability to project or recognize what situation or condition will result from current actions in the near future, to choose between 'positive' (pleasing) or 'negative' (unpleasant) activities and the suppress socially unacceptable responses to certain stimuli. It also assists in the determination of what things are similar and which are different, as well as helps retaining longer term memories from non-task based actions.

These long term memories are often associated with emotions. The temporal lobe's function in the human brain supports this closely related purpose by processing sensory input, storing visual memories, language comprehension, and the creation of new memories.

The cingulate cortex is an integral part of the limbic system in the brain. It further supports these other players through the formation of emotions related to memory and the processing of learning.

Underneath the cingulate cortex lays the subcortical area of the brain. The pathways found here enable quick, unconscious reactions. This means that any reflex you experience, such as jerking your hand away from a hot stove, is a subcortical reaction.

BRAIN FUNCTION IS VITAL FOR A GOOD SEX LIFE
Seeing how important the brain is for healthy sexual interactions, it's pretty much a "no-brainer" that anything along the lines of brain injury or psychological issues (such as depression) will almost always interfere negatively with our sexual responses.

After all, healthy and pleasurable sex is what we all want and this is where Dopamine comes in.

You may have heard of Dopamine, a chemical secreted by the brain that has an immense role in our moods and emotions and it's commonly known as the 'feel good' chemical. It is responsible for the pleasure we experience in relation to certain types of decision making, such as choosing certain foods or even solving mathematical problems.

This 'feel good' sense we get aids us to preplan our movements, aides the brain in filtering out and sorting what smells like what, and sorts what we see, what we hear, and other data that is constantly bombarding the senses.

Dopamine also helps us make certain behavioral choices we use to guide us on our path to achieving our own personal goals. When Testosterone falls below optimal levels men tend to demonstrate more mood-related disorders, despair, sadness, misery – all forms of depression. Good mental health and Dopamine function are therefore reliant on healthy Testosterone levels.

Moving down through the brain structures and working our way south, we come to the spinal cord, another important component of the brain system intimately connected to male sexuality. It's important as it relates to the male erection. The part of the spinal column responsible for erections is located between T11 and L2, the lower thoracic and upper lumbar.

DEFINING TYPES OF ERECTIONS

Here's something you may not know. Not all erections are created equal. There are actually three (3) distinct categories of erections that have been identified. They are defined as follows:

Psychogenic: This type of erection occurs when you have mental stimulus (thinking or seeing something you find sexually stimulating or sensual). It can come from something you see, something you hear, or thoughts that you have regarding something sexually stimulating. Even the memory of a past sexual experience falls into this category. Sexual stimulation brought on by viewing porn is a prime example of erections found in this category.

Reflexogenic: This type of erection is a direct result of touch or stimulation to the penis. Things such as stroking, caressing, or oral sex are known stimulants. (As if you didn't know that!)

Spontaneous: This category of erection comes from some form of internal stimulation. Awakening with an erection, the good ole' "morning wood", is very natural after puberty for most of us.

Yet another example of a spontaneous erection is getting stimulated to erection from the pressure of having a full bladder.

Reflexogenic and Spontaneous erections are both controlled by the nerves found in the lower segments of the spinal cord.

EJACULATION IS A COMPLEX PROCESS

On the same vein, the ability to ejaculate is extremely complex. It requires coordinated activity by the brain, spinal cord, nerves and the penis all working together as a team to make ejaculation occur. If one thing is amiss within the process, it will become problematic at best. This does not mean sexual desire is absent because, as most men realize, sexual pleasure and sexual function are in large part psychological.

Blood vessels and multiple hormones, such as Testosterone, also play a large part in having a healthy sex life. Interference with either of these factors, including those previously mentioned, from your brain down to your spinal cord, will result in sexual dysfunction. You can count on that.

And if that isn't complicated enough, let's talk more about those male human reproductive organs.

This is another intricately interconnected system and every one of these components is regulated by Testosterone or one of the natural derivatives of Testosterone, such as DHT (Dihydro-testosterone) and Estrogen.

All of these work together to help our bodies work. Unfortunately for us, it's not always a fool proof system.

The reproductive organs for the human male include:

- the penis,
- testes,
- epididymis,
- vas deferens,
- the seminal vesicles,
- the prostate,
- Cowper's gland
- ejaculatory duct.

TESTOSTERONE AND THE TESTES

Testosterone is responsible for the maturation, physical growth (increased size, musculature, facial and body hair) and the function of various reproductive organs. After adulthood is reached, the receptors for growth, especially in the penis, are absent. At this point, Testosterone is only responsible for continued function and maintenance of reproductive organs.

The majority of a man's Testosterone, 95% to be precise, is produced by Leydig cells. This rather small, mass of tissue makes up only 2.5% of the testicle. The rest of its volume consists of blood vessels and connective tissues. A rather large quantity of Testosterone is required to produce sperm so the testicles produce proteins in order to keep large amounts of Testosterone in the testes.

Scientists now say that the amount of Testosterone can be up to 100 times as much as found in the blood and the average size of the average adult tactical is roughly 2.0 inches long by 1.33 inches wide. A whopping 90% of this is sperm manufacturing tissue.

ERECTILE FUNCTION/ERECTILE DYSFUNCTION

One symptom brought on by aging, as well as Andropause, is erectile dysfunction. Basically, an erection occurs when sexually arousing stimulus results in a rush of blood flow to the vessels and tissues inside the penis and it thus becomes firm and swollen with blood.

As simple as it may seem, this really is a complex process. We can reduce the complexity by focusing on two chemicals that play a major role in sexual arousal in both genders. Nitric oxide and cyclic Guanosine Monophosphate (cGMP), both of which are responsible for the response of smooth muscle and blood vessels found within the penis.

This increase in blood flow, as well as these two chemicals, is influenced by DHT. The main regulator of these chemicals and DHT are manufactured from - you guessed it - Testosterone. Without sufficient Testosterone available in the body, there is not enough DHT to influence the NO and cGMP to aid in the creation of an erection. OMG!

In the case of erectile dysfunction, there are a multitude of possible causes. Changes in blood vessels that result in less blood being carried to the penis is one possible reason. There could also be problems in the nervous system that result in lack of stimulation of the nerves necessary to produce an erection.

Other major contributing factors leading to erectile problems can be certain medications. Blood pressure medication, SSRI antidepressants, anticholinergics and corticosteroids, could all be blamed, just to name a few.

Hormonal issues like too much prolactin (a pituitary hormone) or low Testosterone (which is very often the case) might be the cause as well. The most reliable indicator of Erectile Dysfunction (ED) is the loss of morning erections.

Outside of the obvious sexual implications, there are many other ways erectile dysfunction can affect men. Those with Erectile Dysfunction have a higher level of depression and anxiety-related symptoms. There are also reports of heightened levels of anger and incidence of personality disorders, impaired social and job function, as well as cases of substance abuse. None of this should come as a surprise when you talk about taking away a man's ability to fully satisfy himself or his partner in the most intimate way.

AGING AND SEXUALITY

It's widely known and accepted that men usually reach sexual prime by the late teens through the early twenties. As we age, a lot of things begin to decrease including:

- Sexual responsiveness,
- Semen volume,
- Interest in sex and,
- Our Testosterone levels.

We also begin to notice that it takes more time to achieve a full erection, and that it takes more direct or intense genital stimulation to sustain the erection, and the penis becomes flaccid sooner after sex. And, let's not forget that regaining an erection again shortly after ejaculation takes longer, if it can even happen at all. Orgasms frequently become less intense as well.

There's little doubt that the aging process has a dramatic impact on our sexuality, mostly due to the decrease in Testosterone production.

As we age there is less of what is called the "luteinizing" hormone, also made by the pituitary gland, to stimulate Testosterone production in the testicles.

At this point, there are also fewer receptive "Leydig" cells found actively in the testicles themselves. This occurrence, coupled with the binding of Testosterone by the blood protein Sex Hormone Binding Globulin (SHBG) or Sex Steroid-Binding Globulin (SSBG) and reduced activity of the Testosterone that does exist (bio-available), makes it more difficult for the male to keep up maintenance.

No man should have to put up with and accept sexual problems due to Andropause and aging with the notion that "that's just the way it is" and there's nothing else that can be done about it.

Fortunately, there are some effective treatments available. The best non-prescription treatment for Andropause we've found thus far that meets our tough standards for product reliability and safety can be purchased at - **http://www.provacyl4men.com**

As a human growth hormone (HGH) releaser, Provacyl™ is an all-natural daily supplement positioned to help millions of men address the symptoms of Andropause, or the gradual decrease of hormone production in men, with a potent and natural blend of herbals, amino acids and nutrients that are clinically proven to:

- naturally increase the male sex drive
- help reduce excess body fat
- increase lean muscle mass
- boost physical stamina
- produce feelings of well-being and positive life outlook

Let's face it, guys are always going to want great sex, look good and feel great. The good news is that with Provacyl™, you can do it without the pain or high expense associated with using synthetic HGH injections. Nothing else comes close.

Provacyl™ has a list of happy clients, produces no known side effects and offers hope to men around the world who want a safe and affordable way to enjoy their golden years.

- Author's Note -

Get Instant Access To This Breakthrough Andropause Solution By Clicking On The Special Risk-Free Discount Link Provided Below…

>>> http://www.provacyl4men.com <<<

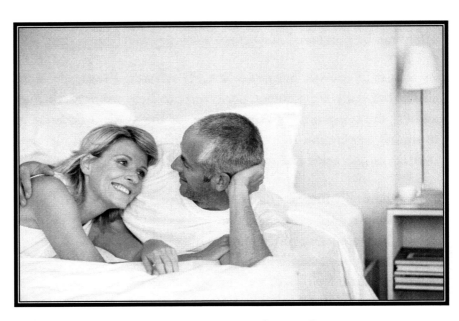

- Enhance Intimacy With Your Spouse -

CHAPTER 5

HOW TESTOSTERONE WORKS

Testosterone is the main male sex hormone produced by the testes. It begins in the womb with production of the hormone beginning in the eighth week of fetus development. As we go through the fetal and embryonic stages of growth, Testosterone promotes penile development, as well as the development of the varied structures involved in producing sperm.

In the early pubescent years (age 9 to 14), Testosterone helps in the growth of testicles. The rise in T-levels during this critical development period early in a man's life is also characterized by acne, an increase in body and facial hair as well as pubic hair. His muscle mass increases and bones strengthen and grow. Sexual maturation and the tell-tale deepening of the voice also are evident.

Later, in adulthood, Testosterone plays a critical role in sexual function and libido; that maintenance job we discussed earlier. And of course, as the male gets on in years, Testosterone also has a hand in hair loss and weight gain, especially around the abdomen, that go along with reaching middle age and beyond.

In the case of the developing male going through puberty, when these characteristic changes are not apparent doctors will usually suggest a number of tests to decide if you have a condition we've touched on before, called Hypogonadism. So Hypogonadism may be indicated when a pubescent male fails to develop normally early in life or a man starts to go through "the change" later in life, having a very close relation to Andropause.

ANDROPAUSE AND HYPOGONADISM: EXPOSED

While Hypogonadism and Andropause are two separate conditions, they can look very similar, especially in the case of late onset Hypogonadism, so it's important to know the difference. To recap, Hypogonadism is basically a drastic decrease in or failure of the male body to produce adequate amounts of Testosterone. Sometimes it is caused by an irregular hormonal stimulation of the testes by other glands such as the pituitary gland. Hypogonadism is believed to be a result of genetic defect, illness or injury that causes the testes inability to perform. That's why it is especially important to protect your "family jewels". A kick to the groin, whether intentional or accidental, is not only extremely painful (and NOT funny), it can have some serious health repercussions.

Symptoms may vary significantly with age of the male as well as the exact cause of the Hypogonadism. Even in the womb, if the male genitalia in the developing fetus is not fully or properly formed by the 12th week of gestation, the diagnosis would normally be Hypogonadism.

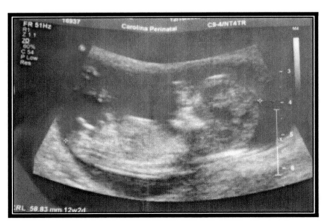

12 week male fetus.

During childhood, boys tend to go into puberty late or even not at all while displaying reduced development of male organs and body hair. Additionally, they seem "small" for their age, while showing low muscle tone, as well as a high-pitched, pre-pubescent voice. When these things appear in teenage males, Hypogonadism is usually to blame.

Actually, the impact of this condition later on in a man's life closely mirrors the development issues in puberty; they just go in the opposite direction. When dealing with adults, the effects of Hypogonadism may materialize in the form of reduced sex-drive, low potency, low sperm production and an overall reduction in body strength.

Your physician will need to rule out any other possible causes for those changes, as an accurate diagnosis of Hypogonadism will require a thorough medical history, physical exam and hormonal study.

Chromosomal examination can also determine the specific cause with blood testing. As scary as it may sound, a simple Testicular biopsy and a standard semen analysis can help determine the status of sperm production. These procedures can also help identify lowered sperm development and evaluates the effect of low Testosterone levels on the individual.

Once an exam has been completed and testing has determined the underlying cause of the Hypogonadism there are several different treatments available. Many forms of treatment consist of Hormone replacement therapy to help fight the effects of low T-levels that characterize this illness.

TESTOSTERONE REPLACEMENT THERAPY IN MEN

At this point, we're pretty clear that Testosterone levels decline naturally over time as men age and that this decline in a crucial hormone is often the root cause of many subtle (and not so subtle) symptoms of the male's version of "the change".

This form of menopause (what we're calling Andropause) may also be caused by Testosterone receptors growing less receptive with age, while bio-available Testosterone in the body diminishes.

The decrease may likely be caused by an increase in that blood protein, SHBG that we spoke of early on. This pesky protein binds with Testosterone, rendering it useless for the multiple, critical functions it is responsible for.

Testosterone replacement may be applicable for the treatment of adult and male youth Hypogonadism. And, scientists often consider that using Testosterone replacement may assist in dealing with the symptoms of a natural declination of T-levels in normal Testosterone producing older men as well.

Testosterone replacement can be done through oral medication, via a simple injection, or by using a patch (transdermal). The FDA approved, about 20 years ago, two types of patches for widespread use. Testoderm and Androderm are both slow release medications that help men with Hypogonadism slowly increase their low T-level through releasing a steady, minute quantity of Testosterone into the blood steam gradually.

However, there are some side effects of Testosterone therapy that must be carefully considered when undertaking this common form of treatment. These side effects often include indications of irritation, aggravation, agitation, and nervousness, plus a more rapid heartbeat, and polycythemia (too many red blood cells), and increase in the growth of the prostate.

Because of this, most physicians highly recommend that you have an annual prostate evaluation by your medical doctor along with a PSA exam (Prostate-Specific Antigen), which is a simple and painless blood test to determine your PSA levels before and after Testosterone therapy to help rule out prostate cancer.

A high PSA is often an indication of prostatitis (inflammation of the prostate), and another exam, called a FREE-PSA will likely be called for to offer a comparison.

Before we go any further, I should address a common question some guys may have; can I use Testosterone therapy to boost my athletic performance? After all, its use is fairly widespread (although taboo) in the world of competitive sports. The simple answer is DON'T DO IT. Using Testosterone supplements in healthy men, in order to improve their performance athletically, or sexually, is especially harmful and here's why:

Testosterone supplement usage may cause some horrid side-effects. Pretend that this is a menu, which of these do you want?

- anxiety, nervousness, depression,
- headaches,
- nausea, and chronic gastrointestinal issues,
- blood clots,
- abnormal bone growth,
- growth stunting prematurely,
- high cholesterol levels.

And, if you misuse Testosterone for a long time, the impact of this is usually the suppression of normalcy in your Testosterone production system. Yes, using it can indeed suppress the body's natural production and T-levels. Now, after reading that serious list of side effects, would you really want to risk it? I hope not.

TESTOSTERONE IN WOMEN

It may surprise you to learn that women also produce Testosterone, in addition to Estrogen. Likewise, men require a certain amount of Estrogen to function normally. As always, the secret is the balance between the two dependent on the primary functions required, whether it's growing a healthy fetus in a womb or producing sperm.

There is increasing awareness that many women experience symptoms of androgen deficiency after either natural or surgically induced menopause.

The pre-dominant complaint of affected women is less sexual desire (diminished libido).

Many women experiencing the clinical symptoms of androgen deficiency and low free Testosterone levels respond well to Testosterone replacement therapy, or menopausal androgen replacement therapy (MART).

However, the effectiveness of MART in relieving these symptoms compared to the more traditional Estrogen and progestin hormone replacement therapy (HRT) remains in question.

Additional concerns are related to the risks associated with developing endometrial hyperplasia and breast cancer when MART is used in conjunction with Estrogens.

The safety profile of MART seems to be generally acceptable when dosing avoids Testosterone levels that significantly impact normal physiological functions in the body.

– KRON 4News – San Francisco – Dec. 3, 2008

Armed with this information, it would be wise to start with smaller doses.

However, only time will tell as they are still evaluating the long term effects of Estrogen therapies at this late date, while studies of androgen effects are still at a very preliminary stage.

Like I said, only time will tell as their use becomes more widely accepted and studied.

For your viewing pleasure we have provided the following chart showing what the normal Testosterone ranges are for a healthy man at various stages of adulthood:

Measurements in European Units (nmol/L)					
Age	Total Testosterone	Standard Deviation	Free Testosterone	Standard Deviation	SHBG	Standard Deviation
25-34	21.38	5.90	0.428	0.098	35.5	8.8
35-44	23.14	7.36	0.356	0.043	40.1	7.9
45-54	21.02	7.37	0.314	0.075	44.6	8.2
55-64	19.49	6.75	0.288	0.073	45.5	8.8
65-74	18.15	6.83	0.239	0.078	48.7	14.2
75-84	16.32	5.85	0.207	0.081	51.0	22.7
85-100	13.05	4.63	0.186	0.080	65.9	22.8

Measurements Converted to (ng/dl)					
Age	Total Testosterone	Standard Deviation	Free Testosterone	Standard Deviation	SHBG (nmol/L)	Standard Deviation
25-34	617	170	12.3	2.8	35.5	8.8
35-44	668	212	10.3	1.2	40.1	7.9
45-54	606	213	9.1	2.2	44.6	8.2
55-64	562	195	8.3	2.1	45.5	8.8
65-74	524	197	6.9	2.3	48.7	14.2
75-84	471	169	6.0	2.3	51.0	22.7
85-100	376	134	5.4	2.3	65.9	22.8

Chart courtesy: http://www.mastersmensclinic.com/male_sexual_function.htm

CHAPTER 6

DIAGNOSING ANDROPAUSE

Now that we've talked about what it is and how it works, let's talk about finding out if YOU may actually suffer from it.

Concerns and issues surrounding Andropause can be handled by your general practitioner and the testing required for accurate diagnoses is extensive but readily available. Your doctor will ask about the symptoms you are experiencing and by now you should certainly understand the importance of being as specific and detailed as possible.

Due to the subtle and highly variable nature of Andropause symptoms they must be carefully evaluated since many symptoms of Andropause are so similar to other possible and common health problems. Your doctor will probably order diagnostic testing to rule out any possibilities other than Andropause and you'll likely need to do a series of blood tests, including an accurate measurement of your Testosterone levels.

I cannot stress this enough; Andropause is not to be taken lightly.

Experts recommend that men experiencing very pronounced symptoms seek immediate and appropriate treatment from a qualified health care professional.

When paired with other symptoms such as weight gain and decreased bone density, other more serious health problems will occur if ignored and left untreated.

Some of these symptoms we've discussed that you should definitely talk with your doctor about are:

- lowered libido or sex drive,
- weaker erections or difficulty achieving them,
- less intense orgasms,
- diminished energy levels,
- decreased strength and endurance,
- joint aches or stiffness in the hands,
- decreased productivity at work,
- loss of satisfaction with life,
- apathy towards things that formerly brought enjoyment,
- depression,
- desire to isolate,
- fatigue,
- falling asleep after dinner,
- urinary changes,
- significant weight gain (especially around the belly),
- hot flashes,
- irritability,
- extreme mood swings,
- insomnia and other sleep disturbances,
- premature or sudden aging,
- changes in hair growth,
- changes in skin quality,
- increased anxiety,
- loss of self-confidence,
- poor concentration,
- memory loss.

ANDROPAUSE AND MEMORY LOSS

Memory loss, is a frightening part of the depletion of normal Testosterone levels, and can be one of the symptoms that is the most hardest to deal with.

It doesn't impact youthful erectile dysfunction patients or those with male child Hypogonadism. This is probably secondary to the effects of the declining hormones that aging men experience which may include:

- Testosterone: total and free Testosterone

- Dehydroepiandrosterone (DHEA) & Dehydroepiandrosterone sulfate (DHEAS)

- Growth hormone and insulin-like growth factor-1 (IGF-1)

- Other hormones including Triiodothyronine, Renin and Aldosterone

    - from Asian Journal of Andrology – **Sept. 3, 2001**

The effect of hormones on memory in older adults has been the subject of investigation for several years. Women's menopause and the hormone effects on memory and cognition are subjects of in-depth research and have been for many years. There is a great deal of medical research data collected showing the vast benefits of using Estrogen replacement on memory and mood.

Memory and cognition impacted by Estrogen must be determined to be a long-term solution, and separate the discussion from any connection with Alzheimer's or any other aging disorder. There seems to be little data linking cognitive changes in males and hormones at this point.

Improving memory could be beneficial to older seniors in their maintaining independence within their own homes before needing care from others in group homes, or with relatives, or assisted living facilities.

IS MEMORY LOSS LINKED TO LOW-T?
We know two things:

1. The total Testosterone level will start declining in the middle aged male, and will continue declining as they age approximately 100 ng/dL declination per decade once they have hit their 50th birthday,

2. Bioavailable Testosterone and free Testosterone decline far more rapidly starting at age 50.

Bioavailable Testosterone levels less than 70 ng/dL or total Testosterone levels below 300 ng/dL are indicative of Hypogonadism.

--from Asian Journal of Andrology – **Sept. 3, 2001**

We've also discussed how Hypogonadism can lead to symptoms such as decreased sexual urge, impotence, erectile dysfunction (ED), exhaustion and lack of energy or strength, and even visible muscle loss, all beyond the cognitive factor.

Again taken from the published study found in the Asian Journal of Andrology – **Sept. 3, 2001**

There was a study, in a population cohort, described as an 'exploratory analysis', wherein Barrett-Connor and their group had looked at 547 men in a community dwelling who were aged from 59 to 89 years old, living in Rancho Bernardo, California.

The team measured bioavailable levels of Testosterone and Estradiol, Estradiol being the most vital form of Estrogen in our bodies.

After blood tests, the elder men were subjected to standard neuropsychological evaluations to check memory and recall, and the status of their cognitive function. After adjusting the results based on patient's age and education, those with high levels of total and bioavailable Estradiol showed to have poor test results on the BIMC (the BIMC measures memory, recall, concentration and orientation) and also the Mini Mental State Examination (which screens cognitive impairment).

Those men who had the higher bioavailable T-levels usually had much better scores on two tests, the BIMC and the Selective Reminding Test. The SRT is used to evaluate verbal learning and memory by using list-learning procedures and several trials).

This study suggests that older men with low Estradiol and high T-levels had predicable better performance when tested on cognition and memory.

There was one criticism of this study, because the blood biochemical markers including Testosterone were evaluated up to 4 years earlier than neuro-psychological testing was done. One more issue was that even though elevated levels of Estradiol were connected to cognitive problems in the elder male, no consideration was taken for any result variance due to subject body weight.

Due to obese men having more conversion of Testosterone in their peripheral tissues, they have elevated Estradiol levels. And, there has not been, at this point, any parallel studies demonstrating a high rate of dementia in the elderly obese male. Finally, the design of the structure of this study – has no basis in proving casual effect.

Verifying Barrett-Connors' great effort, there was another study conducted by Morley and his team and they reported that there was a correlation between age-related cognitive measures, and physical measures and bioavailable Testosterone.

Epidemiological comparisons similar to those just mentioned also indicate that there is a link. Certainly studies like those previously described suggest there is a link; it will be interesting to discover what the impact will be, therapeutically, in those types of cases to use Testosterone in therapy.

Janowsky's team indicated that there was increases in the subject's special cognition, however no improvement in other cognitive areas; no improvement in memory for older men, after 3 months of transdermal Testosterone patches.

Janowsky, however, discovered that subject's working memory improved after one month trial with healthy aged men after Testosterone was supplemented. This study was conducted on very healthy aged senior men who had no history of any prior memory problems. And therefore, this study indicates Testosterone may be beneficial in the enhancement of memory for normal and healthy men. But, so far this study has not been replicated, and therefore all results are considered speculation.

MEMORY LOSS IS KEY TO ANDROPAUSE

According to a study including more than 300 men, the loss of memory is now considered to be an 'established' symptom of Andropause.

In one more study on older male patients, there are descriptions of how the elderly recognize and understand their own aging.

"We performed a non-interventional, cross-sectional study of our own to determine what male patients report as symptoms of Andropause. In particular, we wanted to ascertain if memory loss was a predominant feature," was how the researchers approached this study.

They claimed their hypothesis was specific in that androgens like Testosterone were important in the function and development of visual-spatial and memory abilities. As apparent as these studies are, aging with Andropause, caused by decline in T-levels, is the apparent cause of memory loss in elderly men.

Remember the study on the 300 patients that I mentioned earlier. They were given a questionnaire with 22 specific questions. Also patient demo-graphics, their perception of what Andropause really was, and the possible risks were explained.

Group demographics: Basis of 300+ patients,

- 71% were more than 60 years old
- whites predominated at 87%
- 36% reported memory loss

Loss of memory was the 3rd most reported symptom of Andropause,

- erectile dysfunction (46%) - #1 symptom
- general weakness (41%) - #2 symptom

Statistics indicated that 22% of the 300+ men had diabetes. Among those with Andropause, diabetic patients were more likely to report memory loss.

64% of those who reported the symptoms of Andropause were between 50 and 70 years. (Median age 50-60 years old).

THE DHEA AND DHEA-S CONNECTION

The steroid DHEA (Dehydroepiandrosterone) is secreted by the adrenal cortex. It circulates through the body and DHEA exists both free and sulfate-bound (DHEA-S).

DHEA secretion is controlled by Adrenocorticotrophin and is demonstrated to have Antiglucocorticoid (which reduces steroidal hormones with an antidepressant action). Its mechanism of action and physiological roles are yet unclear.

There are many proponents who suggest that DHEA has a protective impact on the body for diseases like:

- diabetes,
- cancer,
- aging,
- autoimmune diseases.

DHEA secretion tends to significantly decline with age, and decline more with androgen failure. This exemplifies Andropause.

The hypothesis that the decline of levels of DHEA may be the contributing factor to age-related changes in cognition is being looked at closely due to an indication that DHEA and DHEA-S levels drop remarkably as we age. This has led to a suggestion that the progression of Alzheimer's disease may be linked to the undiagnosed lack of DHEA's protective effect. Sunderland's team showed specifically that reduced DHEA-S levels in people who had Alzheimer's.

Carlson's team in Canada specialized in the study of DHEAS levels and its impact on memory in both men and women who were elderly with Alzheimer's. 52 patients having 76.2 mean age were the subjects of this study. Each patient was individually tested with the Rivermead Behavioral Memory Test. They also got a DHEA-S levels checkup.

Those patients who demonstrated higher levels of DHEA-S were far better in remembering names and faces associated by photo, did better in the digit span test and in the Mini Mental Status Examination.

Yanase's group in Japan discovered a decrease in DHEA and DHEA-S levels in dementia patients suffering Alzheimer's or cerebrovascular disease.

Yanase's study only had a few patients (19) Alzheimer's disease. But, Kalmijn's Netherlands team, demonstrated a non-significant inverse, link between DHEA-S and declination of cognitive skills. In this community study using 189 healthy people, they discovered it was basal free cortisol that was correlated to impairment of cognitive factors.

And finally, the Baltimore Longitudinal Aging Study of 883 community-dwelling males indicated that a decline in endogenous DHEA-S was independent of cognitive status and had no impact on cognitive decline in healthy aging men. This study was "longitudinal and elegantly designed with follow-up for as long as 31 years. There were biennial assessments of DHEAS and cognitive status in this study".

CAN YOU IMPROVE MEMORY IF YOU HAVE ANDROPAUSE WITH DHEA THERAPIES?

Most people who know health food supplements realize that DHEA is widely sold as a health-food supplement over the counter and many of the adults over 50 use this supplement in order to restrict conditions related to cognition and physical change.

There have been numerous investigations into whether DHEA and DHEA-S have the reported effect in reducing the cognitive decline in human.

The Baltimore study we spoke of earlier has not been able to support the theory that decline in DHEA-S causes decline in cognitive abilities in senior males, even after 31 years of following up the study with patients.

Carlson's study also failed to prove that DHEA-S protects us against memory decline with aging, with healthy aging men and women.

Wolf's team indicated that after 2 weeks of DHEA replacement therapy there was no visible sign of any beneficial result in cognitive testing of healthy elderly men and women. That study included 40 men who took oral doses of 50mg of DHEA daily for 14 days. Then there was a 14 day period to clean out their systems, and a 14 day placebo in order to compare.

In Wolf's same study, women participants demonstrated they had better performance in cognitive skills in the picture memory cognitive tests after taking DHEA supplements.

And, DHEA supplement therapy did not have any visible beneficial impact, or any measurable psychological or cognitive improvements. Furthermore, Wolf's study is subject to criticism due to design and size, as well as possible confounders in the study.

In France, another study using a double blind randomized design, 280 subjects, all who were healthy and elderly took either a placebo or DHEA. One year later, after 50mg/day, no improvement in cognition was measured.

Notwithstanding this massive mountain of documented research contradicting the DHEA potential for helping, anecdotal patient reports indicate that DHEA improves their memory, at least qualitatively. NIH in Bethesda, Maryland seems interested in discovering more about DHEA as demonstrated by their upcoming grants.

Right now, we can definitively state that the impact of DHEA on cognition is controversial. More studies are needed to determine whether there are any benefits to cognitive skills in the long-run, from long-term supplements of DHEA. Right now, we might make the assumption that there might be a possible link between DHEA, but no proof exists to indicate DHEA is a positive alternative to cholinesterase inhibitor treatment for Alzheimer's.

There tends to be some support for using Testosterone therapy to have a supportive role in treatment of Alzheimer's, but researchers are not clear if the benefit is the direct effect of using Testosterone or merely a side effect from the conversion of it to Estradiol.

More long-term trials are obviously needed.

SADLY, NOT RECOGNIZED/UNDER DIAGNOSED

Even with all this information available, Andropause continues to be drastically under diagnosed, considering it's a stage of life for men. I find this really sad. While the reasons are many, the most prominent issue is clearly the vagueness of the symptoms and their tendency to vary so much depending on the individual. For far too long, men had simply been brushed off by their doctors and made to believe their age was merely catching up to them.

Today the scenario is thankfully changing for the better. Research has often found that in the case of depression the culprit is actually due to hormonal imbalances. Hormones such as Testosterone, DHEA, thyroid, and Estrogen are all impacted. We know that men produce Estrogen in smaller amounts than women, just as women produce smaller amounts of Testosterone. This is a built-in safety device of the body so that hormone levels do not reach dangerously high levels.

Currently, ongoing research on Andropause is focused on better diagnostic blood tests and improved interpretation of those blood tests. In the coming years, it is likely that men 50 and older will be given the option for Andropause screening. This screening could measure hormonal levels since they differ widely according to age group.

There is already a push by the medical field to improve screening for prostate cancer in men over 50, with the use of PSA level testing. PSA (Prostate-Specific Antigen). Other tests currently available to determine Testosterone and other hormone levels are saliva and blood spot tests. Either of these tests can simply and effectively identify hormones in excess or hormonal deficiencies in the body.

In saliva testing, a sample of saliva is taken and analyzed for levels of the following hormones:

- Luteinizing Hormone (LH)
- Follicle Stimulating Hormone (FSH)
- DHEA

- Androstenedione
- Testosterone
- DihydroTestosterone (DHT)
- Progesterone
- Estrone and
- Estradiol

A blood spot test can also effectively test for these and both tests are even available as home testing kits online. One note of caution regarding home testing kits; Testosterone levels often vary from one day to the next. This leaves room for error in testing, so it's important to monitor your levels over a period of time to arrive at an average. The most widely used method of measuring Testosterone levels is the free Testosterone method. While it is widely accepted, blood work should be done prior to 10 a.m. in order to gain peak values.

I would also caution against using them as your only means of diagnosis because of the serious health risks involved in misdiagnosis. Consulting with a professional is always your best bet, especially when your health is at stake.

Remember that blood work should be done prior to 10 a.m. in order to gain peak values. When testing for T-levels in the blood, men should fall well within the range of 300 to 1200ng/dl. Their FAI (Free Androgen Index) should fall between 70 and 100%. If this index is less than 50% the symptoms of Andropause appear.

There is some controversy over what level of blood Testosterone is considered normal in healthy, adult men. The definition of low Testosterone varies greatly.

The general consensus is that two standard deviations below the usual rate of a younger man is considered deficiency. Feel free to refer back to the chart provided earlier.

Regardless, you and your doctor should work together in order to find out what level is right for you. It should be repeated here that seeing a physician experienced in the field of interpreting Testosterone levels is highly recommended. It makes the accurate interpretation of test results much easier, as Testosterone level reading is complicated.

ANDROPAUSE QUESTIONNAIRE AVAILABLE

Another valuable tool to help in your diagnosis process, the Andropause Society offers an online questionnaire using a 1 to 5 severity scale (1 being none up to 5 - severe) for your symptoms as well as a check list portion. The test has been used by doctors in monitoring patients going through Testosterone replacement therapy as well as determining Testosterone deficiency.

Professor Lothar Heinemann, in Germany, is responsible for the development and validation of this test. At the end, the questionnaire offers you the option to share the results with your doctor.

We have provided you with a modified version of the text, in modern language so that it is easier to understand clearly what is being asked.

Andropause: Self-Test

The symptoms of Andropause develop slowly and may be difficult for the male to explain to his physician: exhaustion, depression, anger and irritability, and reduced libido are the first signs that you might have Andropause. With the following test you should be able to determine whether or not you are suffering from Andropause and to what degree you may be experiencing its effects.

We recommend that you print out these pages so you can take the time to complete and assess the questionnaire at your leisure. Then take it to your physician.

Questions –

Read carefully

Answer 1 to 5

1 = never 5 = severe

1. I don't wake up with a morning erection any more. _____
2. I don't wake up with a morning erection any more. _____
3. I am always tired, exhausted and I have no energy. _____
4. I am always nervous, tense or anxious.

   _____

5. I am mostly depressed, sad and blue. _____
6. I am easily irritated and angry or in a bad mood a great deal. _____
7. I have trouble concentrating and my memory is worrying me. _____
8. I have sexual relationship problems with my partner. _____
9. I struggle with reduced libido and lowered sexual
   energy._____
10. I struggle with potency and with erections. _____
11. My skin, especially on my face and hands, is dry. _____
12. I have lumbar spine pain and joint pain. _____
13. I sweat heavily (day or night). _____
14. I am a heavy drinker (alcohol). _____
15. I am always stressed out. _____
16. I am not in good physical condition. _____
17. How old do you really feel, right now? _____
    (put your age here _____ how old you feel as 1-5 above.)

CHAPTER 7

GMOS – GENETIC MODIFICATION OF OUR FOODS

This is a highly technical chapter on the biology of genetically modified organisms (GMO's). When we refer to GMO's from here forward we are talking specifically about the foods we eat. We'll try to make this as interesting as possible because it is a very important subject in this day and age. It's also an important part of the discussion on Andropause, and because GMO's have a direct impact on Andropause we will make these connections obvious so you can easily find and learn the information you need to know to make fully informed decisions about your health.

To clarify, genetically modified foods (GM foods, or biotech foods) are foods derived from genetically modified organisms (GMO's), such as genetically modified crops or genetically modified fish. GMO's have had specific changes introduced into their DNA by genetic engineering techniques. These techniques are much more precise than mutagenesis (mutation breeding) which describes an organism's exposure to radiation or chemicals to create a non-specific but stable change. The re-engineering of DNA drastically alters the building blocks of that organism. Quoted from: http://drugfreeusa.net/index.php?option=com_awiki&view=mediawiki&article=Genetically_modified_food?qsrc=3044

Other methods used to modify food organisms include selective breeding; plant breeding, and animal breeding, and soma clonal variation. These types of modifications have been around for a while. Commercial sales of genetically modified foods began in 1994, when a Californian company named Calgene first marketed its Flavr Savr (also known as CGN-89564-2; pronounced "flavor saver"), "a genetically modified tomato [and] the first commercially grown, genetically engineered food to be granted a license for human consumption by the FDA." (From Wikipedia)

Those who criticize the use of GM foods typically do so on several concerns:

- safety issues,
- ecological concerns,
- economic concerns.

The economic question of GM plants (and maybe even GM animals) interests us as researchers because these sources of food for humans become subject to legal restrictions of intellectual property, by law, whereby the food supply of the world and trillions of dollars are at stake. But that's for another book, and many articles exist online and in university libraries discussing the pros and cons of genetic engineering. Here we only cover GM food, per se.

At the present time there are only two primary ways to produce genetically modified plants that create food, there are cisgenesis and transgenesis. Transgenic plants will have genes from other plant species inserted into them. Cisgenic, on the other hand, are produced through gene combinations found within either a closely are related species, or the same one, in a way such that conventional breeding can still occur.

In the past, breeders and scientists argued about cisgenic modification, although useful for plant modification, is too hard to crossbreed conventionally, and that cisgenic plants must not have the same legal regulations as others GM foods. As an observer, this is not sound reasoning to me.

GM plants begin with their genetic engineering in a laboratory situation, through alteration of their natural genetic makeup. Then the laboratory will test and evaluate the GM plant to determine if it has the desired qualities.

This can be accomplished through the additional of one or more genetically modified organisms with larger plants, and the larger plants already have been modified to contain the gene which was inserted with its protein properties.

Then farmers grow and sell these GM crops as commodities into our food supply in countries that permit the use of GM foods in the main food supply of plants or animal meats.

GMO TESTING

Testing on GMO's in both animal feel and human plant food is a routine requirement accomplished with molecular techniques such as DNA microarrays or qPCR. These forms of testing are based on the screening for specific genetic elements (like p35S, tNos, pat, or bar) or event-specific markers (like Mon810, Bt11, or GT73).

The use of the qPCR is for detecting any specific GMO events through using a specific CaMV (cauliflower mosaic virus). These are included into virtually every GM crop produced today). Their presence is to avoid getting false positives if they received a sample that was contaminated with viruses.

In a January 2010 peer-reviewed paper regarding the detection of DNA and it's extraction in a complete industrial soybean oil processing chain was noted to monitor for the presence of Roundup Ready (RR) soybean: "The amplification of soybean lectin gene by end-point polymerase chain reaction (PCR) was successfully achieved in all the steps of extraction and refining processes, until the fully refined soybean oil. (From http://hdl.handle.net/ 10198/5015)

This process of amplification in the Roundup Ready soybean by using polymerase chain reaction assays with event-specific primers was achieved for all extraction and refining steps. This was true with the exception of any, except for the intermediate steps of refining (neutralization, washing and bleaching) possibly due to sample instability. The real-time PCR assays using specific probes confirmed all the results and proved that it is possible to detect and quantify genetically modified organisms in the fully refined soybean oil. To our knowledge, this has never been reported before and represents an important accomplishment regarding the traceability of genetically modified organisms in refined oils."

What does it mean? Well, basically think of it this way. "Roundup Ready" refers to exactly what it sounds like: these soybeans were modified to withstand the primary chemical in the commercially available "Round Up" weed killer you can buy at your local hardware store. This engineering allows the farmer of these soybean crops to liberally spray herbicides (weed killers) to obliterate all but the desired crop of choice.

When the soybeans were harvested, cleaned (with bleach, no less!), processed (into oil) and the finished oil product tested it showed evidence of the modified DNA. And who knows what that will do to you, how it will combine in your body, once you ingest that product. It just can't be good - and it isn't.

GMO's have been proven to be toxic, not only for humans, but beyond that – they inhibit our own detoxification of our cells. Now, more than ever, it is important that you become well-informed about the food supply we all rely on for sustenance.

Our bodies have a unique make up of enzymes known as cytochrome P450 (CYP). These enzymes also play a vital role in the well-being and health of mammals.

A primary function of these enzymes includes to provide for the detoxification of our cells from being invaded by Xenobiotics (xeno being the prefix given to "strange" or "alien" things) and also for heavy metals within our bodies.

Xenobiotics can also be responsible for the inhibition of the body's normal function by being in competition to win binding sites, i.e. the sex hormone binding globulin (SHBG) that we've been talking about earlier.

There again is mounting evidence demonstrating that it is chemical agents found in a common herbicide used in agriculture that inhibits our P450 enzyme and leads to damaged cells.

The association between CYP enzyme being inhibited and hormonal performance is vitally essential:

> Since CYP enzyme activity also governs cholesterol synthesis and the production of key sex hormones that are crucial for development – it is also a major player in the epidemic of hormonal related disorders in the U.S. This includes dysmenorrhea, endometriosis, uterine fibroids, menopausal abnormalities, breast cancer, uterine/ovarian cancer, male Andropause and prostate abnormalities.
>
> For example, Vitamin D production and utilization is essential for over 2000 genes and is a key player in immunity and brain development. Lowered vitamin D3 levels are associated with chronic inflammation, neuro-developmental disorders, neuro-degeneration, the development of cancer and arteriosclerosis, among others.
>
> GMOs contribute to rapid rise in chronic disease. **From** http://www.foodandrecipe.net/diet.html (Jan. 5, 2007)

Inhibited CYP enzymes leave the liver and kidneys in a frail state whereby they cannot detoxify the toxins or hazards in our body, life and environment including:

- heterocyclic amines,
- polycyclic aromatic hydrocarbons,

- benzene,
- nitrates.

The liver's inability to metabolize the toxins in our bodies then becomes the major factor contributing to cancer development.

Unfortunately, in today's society we have rather high incidence rates of birth defects, congenital disorders, and early childhood development of neural abnormalities, chronic disease and immune disorders. This is now far, far greater than ever realized before in the history of man on earth.

Our toxic world is under suspicion of being at cause. There is already research showing that Glycosophate has debilitation health impact which includes inhibiting the CYP enzyme. This becomes life threatening when we realized the extensive use of Glycosophate residue in many Americans diets. Remember those Round Up Ready soybeans? The main ingredient in Roundup is Glycosophate and it's also in many other common herbicides widely used around the world today.

The problem with the CYP enzyme being inhibited is only one of the many challenges that are involved with Glycosophate use and GMO's in our food.

There are other issues regarding altered sulfate metabolism, and then there is the damage that occurs to the human microbiome (def. collection of microbes, bacteria, viruses, and single-cell eukaryotes that inhabit the human body) - www.bcm.edu/molvir/microbiome). There are chemically-caused environmental damages negatively affecting our body's usage of genetically altered food. Furthermore, the widespread use of GMO's are probably the most damaging thing that mankind has done to themselves during the new world of technology in food.

Sadly, in this world where giant corporations just employ food modification just for convenience sake and advancing corporate profits, foods that are genetically modified are not our only concern in life. There are chemicals at every turn that impact your health, your life, and your T-levels. Chemicals that impact your health, your body and yes, even your T-levels. Yes, everything from the plastic containers that you store your left-overs in to your shampoo bottle!

You might ask yourself, "How the heck can that happen?" The answer is the magic of Plastics. Xenoestrogens are a type of Xenohormone that mimic Estrogen, and is in almost every kind of plastic that is produced worldwide today. Call Xenoestrogens what they are - "mutant Estrogens." In and of themselves, harmless except when ingested by humans and the environment.

Xenoestrogens are highly toxic to you, simply because your body is not equipped with a system to expel Xenohormones. They get trapped within our fatty tissue and it disrupts the natural T-level balance within our bodies. Xenoestrogens practically have the power to essentially turn men … into women.

Want to avoid exposure to Xenoestrogens? – Easy, study about the shampoos you use in your life. Read the labels. Don't buy or consume shampoos or other products containing:

- **Parabens** – Parabens are in the majority of all of the mass manufactured personal care products. They lengthen product shelf life.

- **Sulfates** – Sodium Lauryl Sulfate and Sodium Laureth Sulfate these are certainly in the majority of mass manufactured shampoos today. Those products add foam when you massage your head creating lather. These two sulfates are in car engine degreasing compounds, and the foaming soaps found at typical commercial carwashes. When you massage shampoo into your scalp, they are immediately absorbed into your bloodstream.

- **Propylene Glycol and Polyethylene Glycol** – Years ago I heard of dogs and cats dying on the driveway of their homes because they had licked the sweet-smelling antifreeze fluid that leaked from the car's radiators. Toxic, poison, antifreeze and oven cleaners too, Propylene Glycol and Polyethylene Glycol are in our hair and body, shampoos and more because they stabilize the added fragrance. These chemicals break down the cellular structure causing Xenoestrogens to become more rapidly absorbed by your bloodstream.

Also, rethink the plastic water bottles that you drink from. They are Estrogenic due to their shipping methods. Shipping in containers that can reach temperatures in excess of 140°F (60°C) before it reaches the store shelf, Estrogens get released when the plastic heats up.

Now with that new found knowledge, let's take a look at TV dinners and their plastic trays. Or how about the plastic food containers we use to heat food in the microwave? Sure, they say they're microwave safe -- but are they human safe? Cooking in any sort of plastic is never a good idea because heating releases toxic fumes from the chemicals they are made of.

Your morning coffee is even suspect. If you work in an office, chances are you drink it from a Styrofoam cup or maybe you're a Starbucks loyalist. Hot coffee causes the Xenoestrogens in the Styrofoam to leak out into your coffee. How's that for two creams and a sugar?

While eliminating all Xenoestrogens from your life can prove to be nearly impossible, there is a way to fight back naturally. Here are a few foods that actually fight the absorption of Xenoestrogens. In an effort to improve your health and well-being, be sure to include them in your diet arsenal:

- Broccoli
- Cabbage
- Kale
- Brussels Sprouts

The conifers listed above as well as others are loaded with indole-3-carbinol (I3C), which the body converts into Dindolymethane (DIM).

DIM causes some specific liver enzymes to block it from producing toxic Estrogens and at the same time increases the production of hormones that are beneficial.

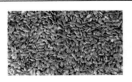 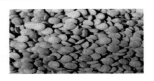 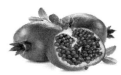

Flax is loaded with Secoisolariciresinol Diglycoside (SDG), which transforms into Lignans (a class of Phytoestrogens) in the body, assisting the body in balancing out Estrogen levels by binding to the same receptors as Xenoestrogens.

Lentils works to purge the body of Estrogen, as they are high in soluble fiber. Consume them as a vegetable or use them in soup and eat them regularly.

Pomegranates are effective in blocking the majority of Estrogenic activity.

CHAPTER 8

THE PROSTATE AND IMPOTENCE

It seems from what we've studied so far, that all the symptoms, and visible signs of a deficiency of androgens is reversible, including the metabolic consequences. The one and simple treatment is a medical method called Testosterone replacement therapy.

Although it's a proven treatment method now available, it's rarely considered by most men. This is usually due to the controversy over the use of Testosterone and its impact on the prostate gland.

As of right now, we don't know much about those effects and what they may or may not do. We do know that men who have abnormally low T-levels usually have small prostate glands. Testosterone Replacement will cause the prostate to grow and potentially reach an ideal size for a given patient's age.

Currently, research shows that using Testosterone therapy will not cause abnormal prostate growth, known as benign prostatic hypertrophy. But, Testosterone Replacement Therapy should never be used with men who have urinary flow restriction (also called outflow obstruction) caused by an enlarged prostate.

TESOSTERONE SUPPLEMENTATION – Be Careful

Scientists do not believe that Testosterone supplements are a causative factor in prostate cancer, however we do know that Testosterone helps prevailing cancer of the prostate grow larger and must not be used with men with cancer of the prostate gland.

RECENT DISCOVERY

Men who live long enough will probably develop cancer of the prostate. It's been shown that almost 80% of all 80-year-old men have cancer of the prostate to some degree on post-mortem evaluation), and this makes it uncertain as to whether Testosterone supplementations can impact older men. To be safe, always be cautious when it comes to hormones and your health.

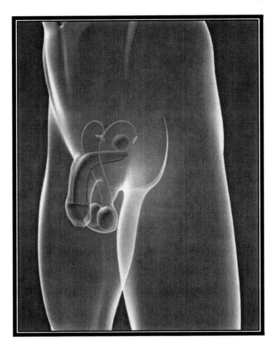

WHAT IS THE PROSTATE?

Before we go any further, a description of the prostrate and its function is in order. The prostate is a thumb-shaped organ, normally about the size of a walnut.

Its sole function is to work as a pump producing and ejaculating semen when a man has an orgasm.

Prostate disease is second to heart disease in causing the greatest health problems a man can face in their elder years. Prostate problems tend to take three primary forms:

- Enlarged prostate (also known as Benign Prostatic Hyperplasia, and sometimes called Benign Prostatic Hypertrophy).

- Prostatitis, which is a prostate gland that's infected.

- Prostate cancer.

ENLARGED PROSTATE

Benign Prostatic Hyperplasia (BPH) is a widespread prostate problem that the majority of men experience; 80% of men will have some enlargement of the prostate as they grow older. The symptom that is most common and most annoying is frequent urination. This can be very frustrating especially at night due to destruction of sleep cycles. Diagnosis of BPH is usually confirmed via digital rectal exam.

BPH is generally caused by poor diet, unmanaged stress, or the circulation of too much Dihydrotestosterone (DHT) which is a derivative of Testosterone, or they just may have excess Estrogen in their bodies.

PROSTATITIS

Prostatitis begins with a basic bacterial infection, and then becomes like an uncomfortable "knot" between the legs. The challenge with prostatitis is that the prostate is wrapped in a "cellular sheath" that makes treatment with antibiotics challenging.

There is also a non-bacterial form of prostatitis, which is unfortunately a chronic problem. The pharmaceutical field has been developing many new medications for controlling non-bacterial prostatitis.

PROSTATE CANCER

The prostate consists of many cellular types, but most cancer of the prostate begin in an area called "gland cells".

Prostate cancer is of the adenocarcinoma type. Adenocarcinoma grows slowly, and is often not detected for a long time, if detected at all. There are, however, less common types of prostate cancer that can grow very quickly.

As noted before, studies show that between 7 to 9 out of every 10 men will likely get cancer of the prostate by 80. The development of prostate cancer in a man is driven by 3 primary factors:

- Heredity
- Lifestyle (especially diet and stress)
- Excess Estrogen

WHAT EVERY MAN SHOULD KNOW ABOUT PROSTATE HEALTH

Testosterone itself is not the exact cause of cancer of the prostate gland. Studies consistently demonstrate that normal and healthy levels of Testosterone actually prevent cancer of the prostate. The cancer risk is related to imbalances in the types of hormones influencing the prostate's functioning.

An increase in risk of having cancer of the prostate can be more related to having an excess of Estrogen in the body. As I mentioned before, too much Estrogen in men is usually related to the existence of unhealthy amounts of fat in their body, especially belly fat. Excess belly fat relates to an enzyme called aromatase, which produces Estrogen from our Testosterone. This is not a good thing for ideal male health.

Occasionally, a portion of the male Testosterone in the body transforms to a more potent form of Testosterone called Dihydrotestosterone (DHT). DHT in excess when combined with Estrogen, can be a contributing cause for Benign Prostatic Hyperplasia (BPH), or an enlarged prostate as was noted before.

But having DHT in the male system is vital for many reasons, particularly, because it's what fuels a man's sex drive. Without DHT, the male human wouldn't have a libido.

In researching the treatment of BPH, we find that some physicians are using medications that will restrict that conversion process of Testosterone to DHT.

The problem with using these pharmaceuticals is that men must make a choice... a choice between alleviating their BPH symptoms and having a libido. What's really frightening is that a large number of men completely lose their urge, desire, and function of sexuality permanently after using these medications. Not a good thing for us at all. And this is the reason that most reputable doctors with a conscious won't prescribe them.

TREATMENT OF PROSTATE PROBLEMS

Unfortunately, the name of the game is prevention. The best treatment is avoidance of prostate problems, through a process of restoration of your hormones to a healthy level. And you can best accomplish this through a healthy lifestyle.

When it comes to the prostate gland, it all comes back to that issue of balance. The delicate balance between Testosterone and Estrogen is critical. Just as women have a lot of Estrogen and just a little Testosterone, healthy men have a lot of Testosterone and just a little Estrogen. Men need that small amount of Estrogen to be healthy, but too much increases the chance of getting prostate cancer.

First, you must avoid getting that belly fat paunch around the midsection, or – you must exercise and diet to lose it if you've got it already. Older, overweight men, carrying extra fat around their bellies, tend to have their Testosterone broken down and converted into Estrogen considerably more rapidly than if it they were at a normal, and more ideal weight.

The other issue is metabolizing the Estrogen. One Estrogen hormone that is produced in the body is Estrone. When it gets metabolized, there are two "safe" paths out of the body: 1) convert it into 2-alpha-hydroxylEstrone, then it can pass out of the body safely, or 2) transform it to 16-alpha-hydroxyl, then it can pass out of the body safely.

But, when the Estrogen in the male body is at cause of prostate gland having cancer, it's due to 16-alpha-hydroxyl being metabolized into something which is called 4-alpha-hydroxyl, a carcinogen. Controlling Estrogen, and helping metabolize Estrone in the 2-alpha-hydroxyl path, are vital to prevent cancer of the prostate.

Take the health of your prostate gland seriously. I now will give you some recommendations for good prostate health:

- Develop good lifestyle habits.
- See your doctor to test and evaluate you, medicate if necessary.
- Take quality vitamin and mineral supplements.
- Consume herbs recommended herein for reducing the risk of prostate cancer.

EARLY PROSTATE PROBLEMS

Physicians have been noticing how men are now experiencing prostate problems soon after their 40th birthday, because during mid-age years men's prostates start to get larger in size and begin closing the opening for their urinary tracts to naturally flow. This describes BPH and it is changing male habits of urinating. Whereby at one point in time earlier in life most men were proud to be able to 'pee like a race horse,' now it's a drip system.

Problems with the prostate can severely impact your health and your sex life in many ways. Perhaps you have to stop whatever you're doing to go and urinate, but more likely as you age there might be a more serious issue with impotence. If you believe you have symptoms of prostate problems, schedule a visit with your physician immediately and discuss it with him.

IMPOTENCE

When we were young, we routinely were awakened every morning to a 'Woodie' or a morning erection. As we get older, there is the rare but occasional loss of erection that occurs. This can actually happen to any male who is post-pubescent, and at any age. Those rare occasions are nothing to concern yourself with because it's usually related to exhaustion, stress or being not in the mood for sex. But, if you are not getting consistent erections – that's, impotence; get concerned and take fast action.

Over the past two decades the ever-changing medical perspective has come full circle regarding the major causes of impotence. This shift has pretty much nullified the age old method of treating patients for ED (erectile dysfunction).

In the past, doctors almost always blamed the psyche of the patient. Even in medical school, professors often taught their students (all the doctors of the future) that psychological factors were always the cause. But all that's now changed!

With men and pharmaceutical companies spending multi-millions of dollars a year for Viagra, Cialis or other ED medications for men struggling with erectile issues, and the extensive surveys and testing that has been done thus far, it's now been determined that over 70% of today's impotency cases are related to some form of medical problem.

Sometimes ED manifests due to psychological effect in life, and sometimes it is related to physical causations. No matter what the reason might be, in most instances there is an easy cure or treatment. Before you go off the deep end with worry, take the first step and go to your doctor to determine the exact cause of the problem. Don't wait because of your ego or you feel embarrassed. Get to your personal physician - be open and totally honest about your problem. The sooner you address it, the sooner you'll be "back in the saddle."

If you are impotent for over 15 days, run some medical tests to check yourself out. Your own personal physician will determine what tests you need. Often ED is a symptom of arteriosclerosis (which is the arterial hardening process); kidney issues, MS, alcoholism or drug-addiction side effects. It could have to do with vascular disease, diabetes; prostatectomy (surgical removal of the prostate), or trauma to the testes (or removal of a testicle).

The tests your doctor runs are specifically to find out if your Erectile Dysfunction is a physical issue or something else. Then further tests can determine if it is prostate enlargement, cancer, impeded circulation of blood to the penis, nerve damage, or hormonal issues. All of these are treatable and you'll be better off the sooner you get rid of them.

Loss of erectile function may sometimes have to do with health problems with other parts of your body.

I suggest that you go and speak with your physician about the issue and get to the cause of it right away. It's important to do so early on because it might be a precursor to cancer of the prostate.

GETTING STRESSED? HELP IS AVAILABLE
Now all this talk about prostate disease, erectile dysfunction, Andropause and the possibility that symptoms may implicate other illnesses, and all the evaluations, tests and treatments, etc. are likely causing you some stress right now. Maybe you're thinking about all the things in your life, including the plastics and processed food that you never considered affecting your health before. You might be stressing about feeling like everything you've done up to this point has got you on a one way street headed straight for big prostrate problems down the road.

Well, stress might be the issue and stress is something that is easy to treat and easy to control. It's well documented that stress affects the body so learn to deal with a problem with a clear mind, without worry and stress. We can help you learn to cope with stress by teaching you some techniques to help you relax, and see things without stress or emotion.

A clear, stress-free mind will allow you to make wise choices concerning your health and well-being. So right now, I'd like you to take a few deep breaths through your nose and fill your lungs with air. Hold that breath ... for a few seconds, and then slowly exhale through slightly parted lips. And, just allow yourself to completely relax. R-E-L-A-X.

Do a few more deep breaths just like the first, and feel yourself begin to relax more with each breath. Imagine the stress being expelled with each exhale.

Why? Because you need to relax and be free from stress to overcome this problem naturally. Taking deep breaths reduces stress, oxygenates the blood, and helps increase the circulation of blood in the body. When you take a deep breath, you are aiding your body in circulating blood where it is needed.

Again, I'd like you to take a few more deep breaths through your nose and fill your lungs with air. Hold that breath... in for a few seconds, and then slowly exhale through slightly parted lips. And just allow yourself to relax. R-E-L-A-X.

Learning to relax, through deep breathing is so simple and it's excellent for stress management and health improvement. I recommend studying yogic breathing for health. I've also provided a meditation in the appendix at the end of this book that you should use anytime you feel stressed.

NATURAL ALTERNATIVES FOR IMPOTENCE
Now that you are more relaxed, I want to offer you some natural

alternatives for treating your impotence. It's a little ironic that some prescription medications used to treat the symptoms of impotence can actually cause it. You don't need to run to get a Viagra prescription, and Viagra is no cure for impotence. Recently, many side effects and even deaths have occurred from using this "wonder drug" which should set bells off before you ever consider taking it.

No longer does any seasoned doctor assume that ED is "all in your head," even though there are times when impotence is certainly caused by some psychological problems. More often now there is a physical causation, and let's take a moment to look at these and some natural alternatives and herbs that can be used for treatment. Remember, if using herbs, be sure to inform your doctor what herbs you are taking. And, if you are already taking some pharmaceutical medication, remind your doctor what you are taking before you start to use herbs.

Common Physical Causes of Impotence

- Diet,
- Smoking,
- Abusing alcohol,
- Abusing drugs,
- Lack of blood flow to the penis,
- Nerve damage or conduction problems,
- Hormonal imbalance,
- other health problems.

All too often, there is more than one problem causing the erectile dysfunction, such as diminished penile blood flow and abusing alcohol and drugs, or another combination effect. Take that into consideration when looking through the list above; if you can tick off two or more of these as potential causes in your own life, you will need to address them in multiple ways.

HERBAL TREATMENTS

Stinging nettle root (1-2 tsp., 5-10 drops it in tincture form or 500 mg. 2x daily in capsules) reduces Testosterone-protein binding to about 10% of prior amount, allowing the access to more free Testosterone for the brain and other receptors.

Avena sativa (1-2 tsp., 5-10 drops it in tincture form or 500 mg. 2x daily in capsules) comes from wild oats straw. I helps released bound up Testosterone also.

Red clover extract has elevated levels of isoflavones genistein and daidzein. These are also in soy products. These natural chemicals are involved with normalizing male sexual function in our later years, but are a preventative for many forms of cancer including prostate cancer.

Muira puama, which is a live plant that originates from the Amazon rainforest of Brazil and Peru, has already proven effective in enhancing the male libido. In South America it has shown significant history as aphrodisiac. This plant can duplicate the activity of the body's natural Testosterone. Men normally will take 1-2 ml. (a dropper full) of the extract in water, 2-3 times daily. Or they might take two 500 mg. capsules. Muira puama takes a period of several months to fortify the system to feel the difference, although some men have reported a change within 2 weeks. Why not give it your best shot, it can't hurt. In fact, Muira puama has no known toxic effect at any dose – and, men usually tolerate it use without problems.

Maca has recently been rediscovered. A Peruvian root, with tribal and shamanic use background significantly improve erection response. It seems that Maca has the ability to normalize male steroid hormone levels including our T-levels, Progesterone and Estrogen to the levels they were at when we were young adults, and therefore restoring our libido.

Dosage for men: is usually around 1,500-6,000 mg or more per day, divided into 3 equal doses. One tsp. of Maca root powder has 2,800 mg of maca root. Add that to one 4 ounces of water, stir briskly and drink three times daily for best result.

Saw palmetto is world famous in the holistic health genre as a viable and effective treatment of enlarged prostate gland. It's become very popular in treatment in reversing an enlarged prostate gland (BPH) especially in elder men. You can estimate that 60% of all men 50 or over are now suffering from BPH and it interferes with sleep and dreaming and also impairs sexual function Saw palmetto used properly can reverse these problems. Saw Palmetto prevents Testosterone from becoming Dihydrotestosterone, the altered form of Testosterone believe to be a causative agent in the BPH. Dose is 1-2 grams of the whole berries, or 320 mg of a standardized extract.

Ginkgo biloba is a very strong vasodilator (causing your blood vessels) increasing circulation to help you achieve firmer erection and improved sexual performance. Like Muira puama, Ginkgo also mimics natural Testosterone in your body.

Black Cohosh Root was discovered centuries ago by Native Americans and is used for helping depression and reducing menopausal symptoms like flashes, mood swings, anger and irritability. The researchers feel that in my reduce bone loss as seen in osteoporosis.

Here's a simple sampling of a few more natural healthcare options you can use, for impotence and symptoms of Andropause. There are many remedies available, from the commonly known to the exotic, including: Vitamin C, Niacin, Zinc, Panax Ginseng, Damiana leaf, Gotu cola, Gokhru fruit, and Elk Antler Velvet.

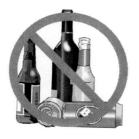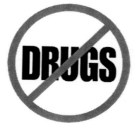

ALCOHOL, DRUGS AND SMOKING

Your physician will probably tell you that you must reduce your alcohol intake, but I will tell you to consider eliminating it all together.

In addition, stop smoking if you're currently a smoker. There's not much else to say about it here and there are hundreds, if not thousands of books, articles and blogs covering these topics and their negative impacts on your body.

Diet is another biggie that must not be ignored, and we're going to devote a lot of focus on it during the next entire chapter of this book.

CHAPTER 9

DIET, EXERCISE AND ANDROPAUSE

The symptoms and change in life that occur with Andropause are somewhat controllable. Preventing serious problems that could arise in Andropause are managed by simply changing your life, including making consistent changes in exercise and nutrition.

There are many ways to treat a health problem after it's been diagnosed. Prevention is undoubtedly the best 'treatment' of all and your diet is a key component on the road to good health.

It's commonly agreed that by eating right, you can improve your health and overall energy level. Eating right basically means using a healthy diet which will enable significant health benefits. The same is true for Andropause; eating healthy foods and living a healthier lifestyle will reap many rewards, including the prevention of serious medical problems.

One of the more obvious things you want to do is reduce your intake of fat. That means eliminate all pork and red meat (except lamb or veal and then only two 4 ounce portions weekly) to prevent further declination in your T-level, the major contributing factor affecting Andropause and all its various symptoms.

There are other things you should completely avoid if at all possible because they are detrimental to rebuilding your virility and vitality. Alcohol is one and we've touched on that quite a bit already.

Then there are all those high-caffeine products that many people consume nearly every day, including coffee, tea, sugary sodas and colas and all those new energy drinks on the market today (like Red Bull). These all deplete the body of Zinc, Manganese, Magnesium (that all play significant roles in the development of osteoporosis) and other important bodily nutrients. Also, be smart and strive to eliminate foods from your diet that have elevated sugar content and are high in refined carbs. Eating them elevates your Estrogen levels, causes an effect to destabilize your levels of sugar in your blood, and destroys some of your body's important nutrients including chromium and all that B-complex vitamins that you've been using to build up your body.

NOW LET'S EAT

You must eliminate fatty foods from your diet, period – no discussion. Good foods for you will be those such as lean meat (not pork, beef and veal), chicken, turkey, lots of avocados, and even eating shrimp, lobster, crab, clams, and other shellfish can serve to enhance sexual function. Fruits and vegetables rich in vitamin B, C, and E also tweak your prostate health and work to help eliminate ED as well.

Here are a few specific foods that are especially beneficial to include or increase usage of in your regular diet:

FISH

Fish is great for your health. Eat plenty of cold-water fish because of their usually high content of omega-3 essential fatty acids (EFAs). The reason for the high fat concentration has to do with being in very cold water for much of their lives.

Now, I know that I warned you about fat intake but these are the healthy fats that your body needs to function well. Examples of cold-water fish include: Tuna, herring, salmon, mackerel and sardines and you can easily find them on restaurant menus or at any local market.

NUT AND SEED OILS

A proper diet aimed at eliminating Andropause must include some unrefined cold-pressed nut oils, and seed oils for your daily eating including flax seeds, walnuts, hemp seed, or pumpkin seed oils.

Because nut and seed oils are high in EFA's your sexual health will improve. Because your body uses EFA's to produce prostaglandins (hormones required for your sexual response). Cooking in those oils is (instead of corn, canola, or other vegetable oils) a very good way of getting the favorable benefits from using the nut and seed oils.

GRAPEFRUIT

Grapefruit is a natural miracle in the fight of the bulge. If you want to drop weight more rapidly, add several grapefruit per day to your diet. Grapefruit is replete with nutrients that you need to increase your metabolism and burn body fat. Red grapefruit is especially good because it contains Lycopene, a powerful anti-cancer agent that works against tumors and cancers because it scavenges on cancer-causing free radicals.

Grapefruit also contains a vital antioxidant called naringenin. Naringenin helps to repair damaged DNA in prostate cancer cells. DNA repair contributes to cancer prevention as it impedes the reproduction of cancer cells." (http://www.3fatchicks.com/)

Grapefruit is also rich in Vitamin C, Vitamin E, and Zinc, and along with many other benefits of these nutrients, all helping to synthesize Testosterone in the testes which is beneficial in addressing many of the problems related to Andropause.

OATS

Eat your oats so you can sew your oats! Oats are rich in Vitamin E releasing Testosterone from the protein that binds it. This makes Testosterone more available to be used by cells that need this hormone. In turn this enhances your libido, builds your strength, virility and stamina, which in turn helps create a more fortified central nervous system.

L-ARGININE: A SUPER DIETARY SUPPLEMENT

There is an essential amino acid that has proven to be very effective for erectile dysfunction, L-arginine produces firmer and long-lasting erections while, at the same time, increasing our desire. L-arginine supplements also seem to increase reduce sperm counts and help in some cases of men being infertile. These supplements open the male to natural remedies in producing nitric oxide, to free up constriction in penile arteries. This is basically how Viagra works. But L-Arginine is must less costly, is 100% safe, and never has killed anyone.

Arginine increases the body's NO levels, and promotes the release of growth hormone that revs up your libido. That hormone helps increase your muscle mass and decreases your body fat, which will definitely make you feel sexier and even make you appear more sexy to your partner.

Dosage recommended: Take 6-12 grams in capsule about 1 hour before your sexual encounter. If this is too much arginine, divide it into 2-3 doses a day of much smaller quantity. And it now comes in a power form to be mixed with juices.

PLEASE NOTE: If you have kidney disease or herpes simplex, avoid taking arginine. Both conditions can be worsened by high-arginine and low-lysine foods such as chocolate and nuts.

All of these recommendations will help you right now, by making a few key changes in your current diet. But if you are comfortable with a more radical change in the way you live, eat and drink, a Mediterranean diet may be the way to go because it fully integrates almost everything we know about the most beneficial diet to improve vitality, energy and stamina; the major issues of concern for someone going through Andropause.

THE BENEFITS OF A MEDITERRANEAN DIET

Have you ever thought that those who lived on a different diet could be healthier and/or happier than you are? Could they possibly live longer or be more virile?

Years ago, the Japanese were hailed for their mostly fish, seafood and vegetable diets for health and longevity.

Today, discoveries from the Mediterranean states indicate that there is something better. Something that will keep you young and virile, or make you feel that way.

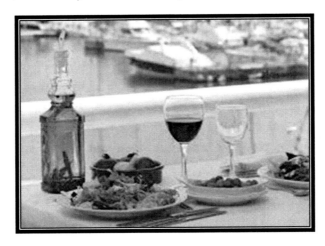

Beyond having some of the most astonishing beaches in the world, physically beautiful people and wonderful year-round weather, the Mediterranean coast has one of the most natural and healthy diets that is renowned for improving longevity while lowering the risk of heart disease.

Take a few minutes to discover the Mediterranean's secrets of their fantastic, exotic, longevity diet, and you can incorporate into your own meal plan.

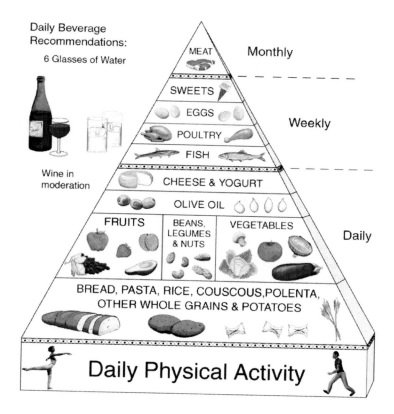

The Traditional Healthy Mediterranean Diet Pyramid

As seen in the illustration above, the base of the pyramid has:

- different grains,
- fresh fruits and fresh vegetables,
- cheeses,
- olive oil,
- legumes, and
- yogurt.

These foods can all be eaten on a daily basis. Next down on the pyramid are the foods to be eaten weekly include:

- eggs,
- fish/seafood,
- poultry,
- sweets.

Those who live on the Mediterranean and those who now follow the Mediterranean diet now eat far red meat and much less often (only monthly) and their fine red wines accompany most dinners, about 1 ½ glasses daily.

THE DIET IS MAGICAL
Fresh fruits, vegetables, and grains

The magic of the Mediterranean diet is fresh fruits, vegetables, and grains on a daily basis. The magic comes in when you realize that these three groups are vitamin and antioxidant rich. Simply when you eat these three, you are helping your body avoid issues with cancer and heart disease. The Mediterranean diet boosts your immune system as well.

Most of the dishes on the Mediterranean diet have copious amounts of onion and garlic that reduce blood pressure and fight infections.

OLIVE OIL
Another important basic food in the Mediterranean diet is olive oil. Those who live along the Mediterranean just love their olive oil. It's the major fat source in their lives with good reason. It's high in monounsaturated fat. That's a 180 degree difference from the fat (saturated) that's in red meat. Olive oil helps reduce the amount of LDL cholesterol which is highly responsible for heart disease. Olive oil also helps us lower our blood pressure and it presents a stomach coating to help us deter ulcers.

Olive oil contains multiple antioxidants to help fight cancer. It's actually quite an amazing food to us to banish unwanted fats.

SEAFOOD & FISH

The Mediterranean seacoast has a great supply of healthy and fresh seafood and fish, and therefore their diet includes fresh seafood and fish recipes which they eat several times a week. Those who live along the coast have thin and healthy blood, due to the omega-3 fatty acid in seafood. This helps prevent blood clot formation and therefore lowers any risk of heart disease.

FETA CHEESE

A generous sprinkling of feta cheese on many recipes is the finishing touch to perfection in the Mediterranean diet. Feta cheese is derived from the milk of goats, isn't low in fat (6 grams in one ounce of Feta), but it's one of the highest sources of Vitamin B12, riboflavin, zinc and calcium. These all help to build healthy bones, teeth and strengthen our immune systems.

NUTS

Mediterranean people generally love nuts. Rich in vitamin E and fiber; nuts are also high in healthy fats, just like olive oil, nuts have monounsaturated fat and that aids in removing LDL cholesterol from your blood. Walnuts and almonds seem to have the greatest impact for lowering blood cholesterol. Nut proteins are high in arginine, and that relaxes you the blood vessels and allows blood to flow more freely. It has multiple benefits for those with ED and Andropause.

DRINK RED WINE

I know I've said that you should avoid drinking alcohol, and that's still my first recommendation but studies have shown some health benefits to certain types of alcohol in moderation – that's the key. The residents of the Mediterranean coast are known to enjoy wine, but they enjoy it in moderation. Perhaps Dionysus wasn't insane when he advised his followers to indulge.

Wine might just be the ultimate antioxidant flavonoid. This is in red wine, and has an anti-clotting effect, prevents the LDL cholesterol from oxidizing in your blood, and more. The recommended dosage is drinking 12 ounces (2 wine glasses) daily. That small amount could help produce some beneficial effects to your health. If you exceed that amount, it just might reverse the positive effects of the red wine.

THE MEDITERRANEAN DIET HAS VERY TINY AMOUNTS OF READ MEAT

Red meat isn't really a desired food on the diet, and it isn't eaten daily or weekly – and that's one reason why the inhabitants of the Mediterranean coast have a far reduced risk of getting heart disease and they also have a greatly reduced risk of Erectile Dysfunction when you compare them to North American men.

GRILLED, BAKED, CHAR-BROILED, BOILED BUT NO FRIED FOODS

Another way that the Mediterranean diet compares much more favorably to the North American diet is that with Mediterranean style cooking – the diet is mostly grilled, baked, or charbroiled, and sometimes boiled. But you will never find fried food in the Mediterranean diet except for a rare delicacy like fried squid.

Whether you prepare your food on an electric grill, or over wood and charcoal on a barbecue pit, making fish on a grill, or grilling your vegetables by first brushing them with olive oil makes for a great meal(s) along the Mediterranean coast – grilling with herbs and spices is just plain … delicious.

SOUP FOR STARTERS

Begin with a light vegetable soap which will allow the pace of the meal to begin slowly, and that way you don't overeat on the main course(s).

HEART-HEALTHY FAT

Comparing the Mediterranean diet to the typical North American diet and you will find that the source of fats in the two diets are quite different. A whopping 40% of the calories come from monounsaturated plant sources in the Mediterranean diet, which helps reduce blood cholesterol while protecting against heart disease and promoting good blood flow for firm erections.

Obviously, the source of fat in most North American diets, however, comes from sources of fat found in fast-food restaurants, and that includes animal fat consumed in meat, butter, etc. none of which is truly healthy for your heart.

EMULATE THE MEDITERRANEAN PEOPLE

If you are serious about improving your condition, I would model my kitchen to that of a Mediterranean chef, and prepare some of their more popular and traditional dishes:

- **Spanish Gazpacho:** this is a delicious cold soup that contains garlic, onions, tomatoes and cucumbers.

- **Greek salad:** start with some lettuce and tomatoes, add feta cheese, black olives, oregano, olive oil, and some red and green peppers to spice it up.

- **Moroccan couscous:** couscous is a grain (semolina) prepared and served with vegetables, cumin, ginger, and garlic.

- **Lebanese hummus:** hummus is amazingly healthy, get some chickpeas mash them with olive oil and lemon juice.

- **Turkish Tabouleh:** here you create a salad from bulgur wheat, onions, parsley, tomatoes, lemon juice, with olive oil.

- **Portuguese grilled salmon:** brush your salmon steak with olive oil and put on herbs and spices, grill on the barbecue.

LIVING A MEDITERRANEAN LIFESTYLE

When you eat the Mediterranean diet, and live a similar and active lifestyle your heart health will likely improve. It's a known fact, proven by years of research, that those living near or on the Mediterranean have considerably better overall health than the majority of North Americans.

Lifestyle is the cause – the Mediterranean lifestyle is one that brings longevity and relaxation. Meals are not in front of TV with family members screaming at each other. A Mediterranean meal is an 'event' where a great deal of time is involved in preparing and cooking the meal. And, a meal is not a 15-30 minute rush proposition. More time is spent enjoying the food during the meal than was spent in the preparation. A meal is a family event to share and enjoy with those you care about.

Extending how long a meal lasts for allows the family to better appreciate the taste of the meal - the extended length of time of a meal also helps one fully digest their meal. And it also discourages any junk food snacking between meals.

Add to that the eating of fresh produce, fruits and veggies, while eating the Mediterranean diet you take in only healthy foods and no processed foods that lack nutritional value.

It's true that the cultures along the Mediterranean are more laid-back than is the case in North American society. And, this reduces stress considerably. Taking a nap in the warmth of sun is a normal everyday thing that people cherish. And this certainly doesn't imply that most people on the Mediterranean coast are lazy and lay around fanning themselves all day.

The Mediterranean lifestyle also requires a judicious amount of exercise to help counteract the fat aspects of the cheeses and nuts found in the diet.

GO MED

The Mediterranean diet is very much in balance with its surroundings — fresh fruits and vegetables are locally grown, and fresh seafood is easily retrieved from the surrounding sea. With modern methods of food storage and rapid produce and seafood transportation, now many people from around the world can feast on this classic Mediterranean style diet — a style of flavor, longevity, and the healthy living of a Greek god.

The primary components of the GO MED program include:

GRILLED, BROILED SEAFOOD, POULTRY, FRUITS, VEGETABLES, GRAINS, OLIVE OIL, FETA CHEESE, NUTS, SEEDS, RED WINE, GAZPACHO, GREEK SALAD, COUSCOUS, HUMMUS

ACCEPTABLE FRUIT LIST

- Apples,
- Apricots,
- Avocados,
- Bananas,
- Blueberries,
- Figs,
- Grapefruit,
- Grapes,
- Guavas,
- Jicamas,
- Lemons,
- Limes,
- Mandarins,
- Mango,

- Melons,
- Nectarines,
- Oranges,
- Papayas,
- Peaches,
- Pears,
- Plums,
- Pomegranates,
- Prunes,
- Raisins,
- Star fruit,
- Strawberries,
- Tomatoes.

ACCEPTABLE VEGGIE LIST

- Beans,
- Beet,
- Black Olives,
- Cabbage,
- Carrot,
- Cauliflower,
- Celery,
- Chard,
- Chayote,
- Corn,
- Eggplant,
- Garlic,
- Green Beans,
- Green Chili,
- Green Olives,
- Green Peas,
- Green Peppers,

- Lentils,
- Onions,
- Lettuce,
- Pumpkin,
- Radish,
- Spinach,
- Watercress,
- Zucchini.

ACCEPTABLE PROTEIN LIST

- Chicken,
- Fish,
- Turkey,
- Soybean Curd,
- Beans,
- Legumes.

ACCEPTABLE DRINKS

- Decaffeinated Coffee,
- Herbal Tea,
- Water,
- Diet Drinks,
- Flavored Soy Milk,
- Lemonade,
- Orangeade,
- Fruit or Vegetable Juices.

ACCEPTABLE SNACKS

- Fruits,
- Nuts,
- Seeds,
- Vegetables or Fiber Bars.

ACCEPTABLE STIMULANT LIST

- Ginseng,
- Yohimbe,
- Horney Goat Weed,
- Damiana,
- Red Wine, in moderation (max. 12 oz. daily).

REDUCE/ELIMINATE LIST

- Sugar,
- White Breads,
- White Flour,
- White Rice, All
- Desserts.

EXERCISE PLUS A HEALTHY DIET HELPS PRODUCE TESTOSTERONE

Another essential part of a healthier lifestyle includes exercise. Exercise and a healthy diet has been proven to boost Testosterone synthesis. This simply means that it improves the ability of Testosterone to combine (synthesize) with other hormones and enzymes to do its important work throughout the body to maintain energy, stamina, emotional balance and all the other things we've been talking about. It appears that studies have demonstrated that you increase your T-level back to normal through regular exercise.

You may already belong to a gym and use their facilities on a regular basis, or you may have your own equipment at home and workout 30 minutes to an hour a day. Maybe you have a regular jogging schedule or ride a bike 10 miles or more three days a week. That's great and if you are doing this, it's adequate for the program. Actually, it's beyond adequate – it's super fantastic!

If that's not you however, we have some minimal exercise requirements to suggest so let's make this as simple as possible.

Our minimum requirements are as follows:

1. Walking: Brisk walking 15-30 minutes after each meal. Walking with another is great, but you must walk after every big meal to activate the body's recuperative powers. Or,

2. 30-45 minutes of Yoga exercises, once in the morning and once before sleep. Or,

3. 30-45 minutes of swimming in your pool once a day.

These are minimum exercise requirements that can help get and keep you in better shape for the sake of your improved overall health.

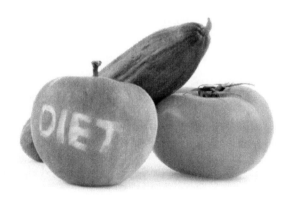

CHAPTER 10

LIVING WITH ANDROPAUSE & TREATMENT

Andropause and its symptoms not only can affect our lives but also those loved ones around us. It can be especially hard to be the spouse, child/children or friend of someone suffering from Andropause. Symptoms like irritability, lack of energy, depression, increased anxiety, mood swings, anger, loss of concentration, and memory loss can put a strain on family life.

It can get stressful at times, so try to be supportive and understanding which is really the most one can do.

MOOD SWINGS

For the spouse of a man experiencing Andropause, one of the hardest things to do is cope with the dramatic mood swings. It's startling to watch someone you've been married to for so long suddenly change into someone you hardly recognize. The irritability and mood swings may be one of the hardest symptoms to handle. Molehills quickly become mountains and causes for major arguments.

These mood swings can leave both parties feeling hurt, angry or lost. It's important to re-assess the situation and handle everything in a calm manner. You don't want to do anything that might cause the anger or irritation to escalate. Remember the deep breathing exercises in the previous chapter? This would qualify as a stressful situation that this method of relaxation can really help to diffuse.

DEPRESSION

Depression isn't easy to handle either. It leaves you feeling unhappy and dissatisfied with things the way they are, because you may have lost your taste for the things you used to love. Depression can lead to isolation because you either don't feel like talking about your emotions or you don't want to bother others with "your problems". It can be extremely difficult to break a cycle of depression alone so you'll need to have the presence of mind to allow others to help you. This next section is for them, but you should read it too.

INSTRUCTIONS FOR YOUR FAMILY

Here we need to try to lure the man who is struggling with Andropause out of isolation and into fun activities and encourage family time together. But, this can be tricky.

It can be especially hard to explain to the children why Daddy doesn't seem to be himself lately. It's important to reassure them when your spouse becomes irritable, forgets things, and lacks energy.

Of course a lot depends on the age of the children; where small children simply cannot understand the concept of Andropause, most teenagers should be able to. In the case of smaller children, it's best to stay calm and tell them things such as:

"Daddy is having a bad day, it's nothing you did."

"Daddy is just very tired lately, I'm sure he'll play with you when he feels better."

"Daddy has a lot of things he's thinking about, maybe he'll have time later."

No man wants his children to fear or hate him, especially when he is not able to control what's happening. Reassurance, comfort and explaining in words they can easily understand is the best way to handle your children when it comes to your spouse's depression.

It's especially important to talk to your spouse. As hard as it may be, you must not simply leave him alone because he may not be able to pull himself out of it on his own. Don't give up and keep your voice calm and your words positive and encouraging. Try to empathize with what he may be experiencing and its okay to ask him to describe it in detail.

THIS CAN'T BE MY BODY DOING THIS

One thing to consider is that when you are going through Andropause, it's not uncommon to feel as if you're living in someone else's body. Women have been warned about menopause and it's symptoms for years, from their mothers to their grandmothers and aunts.

Most men haven't necessarily had this foreknowledge and the sudden change and threat to our manhood can be very daunting. Even with the cultural changes and new acceptance of a man's vulnerability and humanity, there's still a pervasive stereotype of masculinity that says a man must always be strong and not show emotions as we handle our problems alone. It's that long-cherished ideal of 'manhood' and machismo that often sets us up for the suppression of emotions which lead to isolation and depression. **Here's how we need you to help us:**

1. **Talk to us about it.** The majority of us aren't really in the know about what's happening to us and our equipment. It's amazing what a little support can do; reassurance that we're not alone in this. Do research with us so we both know what to watch for.

2. **Guide us to a doctor.** The appointment maker and keeper in most households is the wife. She knows who has an appointment, the time, date, and the all other bits of information. Make sure we know Andropause is

something we can and should discuss with our doctor; that it's something many men discuss with their health-care providers. If reason doesn't work, just show us the numbers and facts because men are more logical and analytical whereas women are more cerebral and intuitive.

3. **Offer us extra support and compliments.** Women often feel less attractive and less womanly during menopause; men are no different in dealing with Andropause. We're beginning to show our age, gaining our father's bald spot and round belly and losing our muscles and memory. Where women chat with their friends about menopause, Andropause is never a comfortable topic of conversation among men. Go that extra mile to reassure us that you still find us desirable. Seduce us. The knowledge that you still see us as the man you fell in love with can go a long way and allows us to keep our self-esteem intact.

YOU ARE NOT ALONE

Andropause can be a very trying time in a man's life as it often makes our close relationships strained and difficult. The realization that you're not alone should be of some comfort. The Hypogonadism in Males (HIM) study found that 38% of men older than 45 years old tested positive for low Testosterone.

It's understandable that men panic when their bodies begin changing and many don't understand that lower Testosterone levels can impact them in such a way. After all, a man cannot see his Testosterone declining but he can certainly see the physical effects of this decline on his body.

It's important to understand just how important Testosterone is. It empowers a man's sexual desires, it fuels his need to protect his family from danger and it's a large part of the lens through which he views the world. That's not to mention all the other bodily functions and responses it affects. Andropause strikes us at the very core of all that defines men as men.

THE TWO MOST IMPORTANT THINGS

Two things to consider when trying to help your body in dealing with low Testosterone levels are watching your weight and avoiding Estrogenic compounds. Watching your weight seems to be the staple for most health solutions. What really brings it home is looking at the statistics on how overweight we have become as a society in the past century.

Between 2011 and 2012, a whopping 40% of middle-age adults in America were deemed obese. The enzyme aromatase is responsible for converting Testosterone into Estrogen and in some men this enzyme is clearly more active due to where this enzyme thrives – in excess fat. The greater the amount of adipose fat tissue means that there is more Testosterone that is being transformed into Estrogen and so on. It's a never-ending process unless you lose weight in an effort to break this cycle.

Avoiding Estrogenic compounds in your household is the second most important thing you can do. As we age, the Testosterone to Estrogen ratio begins to fall and additional sources of Estrogen further upset this delicate hormonal balance that brings on and aggravates the symptoms associated with Andropause.

If this sounds familiar that's because we've talked about it in earlier chapters and it's so important that it bears repeating here... plastic packaging, personal care products, and antibiotic or steroid raised meats and dairy products are filled with endocrine disruptors and Xenoestrogens. Men and women should both avoid them to be sure to avoid an increased risk for cancer.

If you can, choose organic corn fed, or grain fed animal products. Also – avoid plastic containers, be careful with your personal care products – make sure everything is paraben-free and free from other chemicals that are detrimental.

Simply have less exposure to toxins. And being more aware of these in our lives helps not only the man dealing with Andropause but also improves the health and well-being of the whole family.

IT'S A FAMILY AFFAIR

Getting the whole family involved in the treatment process can help bring everyone together in a more supportive way. Making it a group learning experience and sharing information can possibly bring a troubled family much closer and strengthen the bonds that will help you all enjoy a richer life as a family unit. Be creative about it; it might actually be fun.

Why not challenge the kids to a "scavenger hunt" for Xenoestrogens in the home? If they're old enough, it will help improve reading skills, develop awareness about their own health issues and teach them greater responsibility.

It may even provide them with a boost of self-esteem, knowing that they are invested with such a responsibility (once you get past their initial resistance to change). They are taking charge of the family's health and helping you through a difficult life challenge.

If your spouse loves to cook, why not challenge them to create a new dish from the Mediterranean diet or some other healthy eating regimen? It might be fun and very interesting to study different cultures as they relate to healthy eating habits.

Research a new or ethnic restaurant in your community and take your family out to dinner there as a reward. Think outside the box!

These are just a couple of suggestions and whether you try them or not, the point is that including every member of the family in the process of modifying to a healthier lifestyle gives them a vested interest in YOUR health concerns, as well as their own.

It will naturally encourage the emotionally supportive environment needed to cope with the challenges of Andropause. And that level of support will reduce isolation and give you a greater chance of success at improving your quality of life as you all learn to live with, and lessen the impacts of Andropause.

PROVACYL: ANDROPAUSE TREATMENT

You may recall that this recommended product was mentioned earlier, but it's worth repeating here again. The best non-prescription treatment for Andropause we've found thus far that meets our tough standards for product reliability and safety can be purchased at this website - **http://www.provacyl4men.com**

As a human growth hormone (HGH) releaser, Provacyl™ is an all-natural daily supplement positioned to help millions of men address the symptoms of Andropause, or the gradual decrease of hormone production in men, with a potent and natural blend of herbals, amino acids and nutrients that are clinically proven to:

- naturally increase the male sex drive
- help reduce excess body fat
- increase lean muscle mass
- boost physical stamina
- produce feelings of well-being and positive life outlook

Let's face it, guys are always going to want great sex, look good and feel great. The good news is that with Provacyl™ you can do it without the pain or high expense of synthetic HGH injections.

- Special Note -
Get Instant Access To This Revolutionary
Andropause Treatment By Visiting...
>>> http://www.provacyl4men.com <<<

CHAPTER 11

ALTERNATIVE TREATMENT METHODS

MEDITATION FOR STRESS MANAGEMENT

We utilize a medically approved stress management technique, meditation (for stress management) to prepare you for another, more powerful technique; hypnosis for Andropause and Erectile Dysfunction. This will impact the organs and glands of your body in order to produce more Testosterone to circulate through your body in the proper amount for a normal and healthy sex life.

We start with a meditation instruction to guide you to your own personal place where you can experience inner peace and serenity. From there we move on to a healing meditation, and then into the hypnosis.

YOUR OWN PLACE OF PEACE AND SERENITY

Finding your own place of serenity, where you can be free from the stresses of life or tensions of the day, stimulates your imagination and feelings. The result of this process is endorphin stimulation - giving you one of the most peaceful experiences you've ever imagined. Record the italic type below as a meditation...

Visualizing yourself in a peaceful scene can considerably deepen your level of relaxation. You can also use this visualization exercise any time as a quick escape from anxiety and stress.

You can also handle any level of stress in your life with the meditation, and the self-hypnosis that follows, but, let's hope you don't have to.

Let's give you the 'place of serenity technique' right now.

I'm sure at some point in your life, or at some time during childhood, you either visited, or saw a movie that had some absolutely beautiful scenery. I want you to take a moment to remember it, see it as a movie in your mind, the colors, the sky, the earth, the scenery, the air quality, the quiet peacefulness.

Imagine what it would feel like to be there, in the scene, with no one else around, there are no cars, no traffic, not even roads, no one but you and nature and the sun and the sky, and the moon. You can be at any place you want. Even in one that is imaginary with purple sky, red moons, and white earth, if you wish. Create your own, where it is peaceful to YOU!

Other people's popular scenes include a quiet beach, calm lake, or wooded area. Other possibilities: sitting by a fireplace, or floating on a cloud.

Make sure you visualize the scene in detail so that it completely absorbs your attention. Once you have created your peaceful scene, you can return to it after doing your meditation or self-hypnosis exercises, or even imagine yourself there while doing deep breathing, or any other time during your day.

LET'S NOW ENTER THE HEALING MEDITATION
Now that you have your peaceful place of serenity in mind, position yourself in the semi-lotus position, sitting cross-legged and fingers in the mudra pose, like the image that follows.

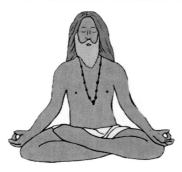

And this is the meditation. I suggest you record it in your own voice – speaking slowly, carefully, and play it back to yourself once a day. It's long, and you'll feel fantastic when you assume the position (semi-lotus) and listen to the audio that you make for yourself. Here are the words:

Get comfortable either sitting up in a chair with your back straight and your feet flat on the floor, or sitting in a cross legged (semi-lotus) position, and close your eyes. And, for a few minutes, just allow yourself to focus on your breath. For the next few minutes, just focus on your breathing. To the best of your ability, feel your lungs breathing in and out...just sense how they feel. Be aware of how they feel while now while you are inhaling and filled with air, pure clean air that you are inhaling, healing purifying oxygen going into your lungs and oxygenating your blood carrying healing energy to every part of your body. And, now see how they feel after you have exhaled your breath and all the carbon dioxide has left your body. You feel calm and pure. Calm, cleansed by pure air, and pure.

Just know that when performing the healing meditation, there's no right or wrong way of doing this -- you are already doing this perfectly, right now. So, draw in another deep, deep breath and feel the lungs filled.

Whatever you feel at this level is just perfect for you. All you're doing now is relaxing, that's fine, just relaxing is great because it's reducing stress and tension, and you are finding that you have nothing to worry about. Worries come to mind, and you no longer react to them.

Just like a balloon, worries float away into the higher atmosphere and then pop and is GONE. As you will see, worries just begin to disappear because you no longer react, you are calm, clear and detached, no matter what you think. It's okay. You'll get through it with a clear mind and without emotional reaction.

If a worrisome thought or any thought comes to take your focus away, just take a deep breath, listen and understand the meaning of my words.

You now realize that now is not a good time for you to be thinking or worrying about anything in life that might, could, should or would; happen in an 'what if' situation, or in any situation in your life.

This is your time, to just let go, let your head down, and for a very short period of time, you can completely relax every part of your body. You know that by always being in control, you can feel at peace and at ease in this, your time of meditation.

Now, again, focus on your lungs. See them in your mind's eye. Visualize them filled with pure, clean air, see them when they are empty. See how relaxed you are feeling. And if your mind drifts away from your lungs, just bring your focus slowly back to where you need to be - on your breathing.

You have done nothing to be worried about, all that you do now and from now on is going to be positive and successful. And, if you can currently hear the sound of my words just follow them. And, if you are so deep that you don't hear my voice, that's okay. Your subconscious is receiving the message, loud and clear, in every word that I say. You hear and understand everything that I say.

Now, in your mind's eye-- just in the center of your forehead - in the center of your brow, you can see a word totally illuminated in retro neon...and the word is visible, it says R-E-L-A-X.

Just relax a little more and see the word RELAX now visible about a foot away from your eyes. And the word RELAX is quite visible. You see it inside your mind's eye, clearly, so just relax.

Close your eyes and draw in a deep breath. While exhaling, say the number three (3) to yourself, three times mentally/silently. Then, slowly calm yourself and concentrate on the top of your head, your scalp. Tell your scalp to relax. Give it a few seconds to begin relaxing. Feel relaxation beginning right now at the very top of your scalp. Relax.

Then relax your forehead. You may feel, during this process, a little tightness around your forehead, or your head. Do not worry, it is the feeling of tingling that may follow the tightness that indicates the beginning of intuitive ALPHA/THETA brainwave production and accessing of the sub-conscious mind.

Now relax your eyes and your eye muscles. Give yourself a few seconds to let that happen. And, in the meantime, just keep breathing deeply and relaxing more and more and more.

Relax your jaw, open your mouth slightly to let the air easily come out of your mouth when you exhale. Then, relax your throat internally and externally.

Relax all the throat muscles and the back and the neck. Give yourself a few minutes to let this happen.

Now relax your shoulders. Let go of the tension. Release the muscles; let the feeling of deepening relaxation enter the shoulders and upper back as you become loose, limp and relaxed. Let the relaxation go into your chest and into your stomach muscles.

Permit your stomach and chest muscles to become looser, limper and much more relaxed. Give yourself a few minutes to really relax these areas. While you are doing this allow the relaxation to enter the upper arms, elbows, forearms, wrists, hands, and fingers. You must relax... relax... relax.

Then relax the hips and buttocks...all the muscles all the tendons, and all the ligaments. Relax the thighs and the hips, totally, until completely relaxed. Relax the calves, the ankles, the soles of your feet and your toes.

Draw in another, deep breath... and mentally say to yourself the number two (2)... three times. And as you do so, just imagine that there are tiny little zippers at the ends of your toes and fingers ... and feel them open and let out all the tension, all the stress, all the worries, all your problems, and just let yourself go. As you exhale all the negativity that you have felt leaves your body. Take a few minutes to breathe deeply and let all the imperfections leave your body.

Take in another deep breath, and mentally say to yourself the number 1— three times.

And as you do so, just imagine yourself in a beautiful nature setting, your own place of serenity. Be there and talk positively to yourself --- this is your own Serenity Place.

ALLOW THE HEALING IN

Imagine that there is a white light surrounding your body, it is the whitest light you've ever seen. It is around your toes, around your feet and it causes you to relax. It enters your toes and relaxes every muscle, every tendon and every ligament. It relaxes every nerve and every nerve ending.

Feel this white light relaxing energy as it moves upward into the soles of your feet relaxing your feet. It causes you to relax every muscle, every tendon and every ligament.

Feel it relaxing every nerve and every nerve ending.

(Then you would continue with various parts of the body, i.e.: Ankles, Calves, Knees, Thighs, Hips, Buttocks, Lower Back, Stomach, intestines, Mid Back, Chest, Upper Back, Shoulders, Upper Arms. Elbows, Forearms, Wrists. Hands, Fingers, then up to Neck, Throat, Jaw, Eyes, Eye Muscles, Forehead, and Scalp.)

If you feel you need to get further relaxed and a deeper induction, imagine you are sinking into a bed of clouds, and if you feel that you need additional focus to deepen your meditation, you can slowly visualize a number appearing in your mind's eye. A number that will appear one less, with each downward number I count, as you count along with me slowly downwards from 100 to 1. You should also time this counting to coincide with every breath that you exhale. (With practice you can use a smaller number as your starting point, 25 to 1, 10 to 1, 5 to 1, 3 to 1 ....)

Remember, you are not trying to go to sleep, you are relaxing into a lightly altered state of meditation. You'll just feel a progressive deepening that many people analyze after they've experienced the meditation.

With repetition and practice you'll realize that it is much easier and faster to reach deeper levels of meditation. Now, focus on ... Jesus, Buddha, or Krishna, placing their illuminated hands, their healing hands on you head and you begin to feel a little tingling sensation. From that tingling you imagine the white light of the Source of all life, God,

is entering. The tingling sensation is breaking the tension down and is disposing of the feeling. The area now feels warmed and healed.

Now, focus on another area - do the same technique until it feels warmed and healed.

Now relax every part of your body until you feel totally relaxed. Feeling that relaxed in your body, you might surprise yourself how good you already feel. Everything is ok, nothing that you do is wrong.

And there's that word RELAX shining out there in your own inner conscious mind, in your mind's eye just behind your forehead at the same time. And you may be surprised at how relaxed you really are. And now you see a doorway to meditation, and if you want to, you can go through the door and you walk through, and -- you can see yourself on a beautiful, warm, comfortable beach with a beautiful crystal clear sky, and a turquoise blue ocean with calm waves.

Everything around you is calm and very relaxed. And you feel the warming of the sun over your body, and you relax more and more and more. You sense a comfortable slightly cooling breeze over your body with the warmth of the sun above – and you relax. You are at peace with yourself, the world, and everyone in it. You hear the waves of the ocean in the background. It sounds like the inner peace that you've always desired.

Feel the warm sand underneath your feet, it's the perfect temperature – just how you like it. And you look behind and see this enormous white sand beach and it looks just wonderful.

As you relax here at the beach, you can remember yourself when you were much younger, smaller, and you were very happy and very relaxed and content at a beach or park or lake. Now, while you are here, recall how content and secure you felt. Feel all that content, that happiness, that security and that carefree emotion. Know that from this moment forth – this is you.

If you happen to hear any noise, it just begins to fade into the background making you relax more and more. And you can recall this memory of feeling happy and content at any time you wish – because it's yours, your own feeling in your subconscious memory and it's easily recalled whenever you desire it.

Now, visualize yourself at the beach again, but this time as an adult... you find a beach blanket, with a comfortable folded beach towel, so that you can lay down with the folded towel as a pillow under your head. So just lay down on your back, your face towards the sun, eyes closed and feeling how safe and secure you are right now.

And now you are surrounded by a golden bright white light. This light covers your entire body while all your normal body functions take place – just breathe in normally – open yourself to the light -

and that golden bright white light combines all the healing powers that exist in this Universe, and all of the healing powers that are now within your own body, plus any and all of the healing powers of any medications you're currently taking or any form of natural, nutritional, herbal, or dietary treatment that you are now using... and that golden white light can go to any area of the body that we ask for it to go, and you ask it to go there now.

Now, begin to visualize any part of your body needing to be helped with this healing light. And I want you to direct the healing light to go directly to that part of your body that needs help. Now surround that part of your body, and any other parts that are in need of help simultaneously. Be aware of the golden light surrounding that part of your body as it combines all of the healing forces of the Universe, and all of the healing power in your body and mind, and all of the healing power of any medication that you're taking and any other healing modalities you are using. It's an extraordinarily strong healing power. And cells are weak or weird they are immediately healed, or are immediately replaced by new healthy ones. You can direct the golden white light to heal any area of your body to improve your overall health -- and to do anything you want it to do. The golden white light is a powerful, vital, revitalizing and rejuvenating force that totally transforms your health and well-being for the better.

Consciously, you envision that the golden white healing light is surrounding any areas where you are not as healthy as you would like to be. And you now can see how this light is bringing the endorphins to work in that area, healing, healing, removing all problems occurring in that part of your body.

Simply guide the healing light to do what you need it to do – it belongs to you, it is yours. Now sense it going where you desire it to go. Feel it there, and by communicating with it you can take charge of your body.

And now before we close this session, I want you put your index finger and your thumb together in the OK position. When you do that you automatically intensify your level of mind, you will instantly and automatically enter the alpha level, or deepen from the alpha to the theta level. During that time frame, your body will instantly and automatically recall the wonderful experience that you are having and which also causes the body to instantly and automatically heal itself, every organ, every gland, and each and every cell.

Now, I will remain silent for a while, and you will want to feel that golden healing light, again – even more powerfully doing all the things you desire for it to do. I will be silent for a few seconds so you can see and feel the light at work. I'll be silent, starting now.

[Pause 60 seconds]

Now, feel that the healing golden white light still remains in your body and travels with you throughout life. It's a powerful force, and it enacts all the positive power of the Universe to help you heal – and you heal. This is completely under control and command, now and always.

Now see yourself walking along the sand. Visualize yourself free from any physical issues, your body and health are perfect and you can challenge anyone your own age because you have absolutely no aches, no pains, no problems whatsoever – you are perfectly healthy.

And now that you're feeling that golden white light, you can call on that healing light that is within you at any time. You call on that healing golden light, at any time you desire, without upsetting your schedule or your life – it's that easy. You simply say, I call upon the golden white healing light – and it is there for you.

In a moment you'll awaken, feeling completely alert and feeling much better than when you started – feeling much, much better.

And now you may open your eyes at any time feeling completely alert, awake and aware.

Congratulations, you have now successfully accomplished a guided healing meditation. It would be best if you could do that meditation once a day for 7 days, using your recording. And then – once a week, on the weekend. This meditation will reduce and eliminate stress and begin the natural and automatic healing of your body and you direct it to do so.

HYPNOSIS FOR ANDROPAUSE AND ED

I got this for you from a friend who is a medical hypnotherapist, and all I can say is … it's like chicken soup – it can't hurt.

Recent medical verification has indicated that hypnosis is a valid treatment for stress and for helping the body prepare for and heal from surgeries. The British Medical Association approved its use over 100 years ago, and the American Medical Association, more than 50 years ago. So, why not give it a shot? It can't hurt.

Do this at home – this is not ever to be used in a moving vehicle or while using heavy equipment. It will cause you to close your eyes and lose focus. NOTE: DO NOT USE WHILE DRIVING.

ASSUME THE POSITION

You can use the same position you did, as in the diagram, for meditation with your spine erect and your fingers in the Mudra position (looks like the Okay symbol). Or, you can lay down on a sofa, or if you prop your head up sufficiently, you can lay in bed or on the floor. If you are fortunate enough to have a recliner (chair), get in and position yourself for comfort.

Record this script below, slowly, as you did for the meditation, and play it back to yourself once you've assumed the position and loosened any tight clothing.

Lie down and relax on your couch or bed, or sit comfortably in a reclining chair. Allow your hands to rest in your lap or rest gently by your side. Now let us begin…

Take three deep, slow breaths, first - in, in, in hold it.....

Slowly exhale and relax...

And draw in another deep breath ... in, in, in hold it.....

Slowly exhale and relax...

And now the last deep breath - in, in, in hold it.....

Slowly exhale and relax...

Each time you inhale while using this program you will focus on filling your lungs with clean fresh air and allowing yourself to hold it, and then exhale and relax.

And as you do so, all the tension leaves your body and you feel so much more relaxed and at peace, relaxed, and at peace.

And with each breath you take you go deeper and d-e-e-p-e-r into the deepest, soundest level of relaxation that you have ever experienced. All the sounds you hear just fade into the background as you go deeper and deeper into the deepest realms of complete and total relaxation that you have ever felt.

Breathe deeply. Allow yourself to relax completely. With each breath you relax more and more, deeper and deeper into a very deep, deep, hypnotic, sleep, deep, deep, asleep.

As your body relaxes, your mind is alert and aware of every word I say. Relaxation is a beautiful experience that you enjoy, and love experiencing daily. By relaxing, you're creating a powerful, alert, and aware state where making changes in your life is easy – so very easy to achieve. In a moment we are going to take a mental journey in order to practice some skills that you desire to learn.

As you learn you will be able to take greater control of your mind, greater control of your thoughts, and greater control of your body. In the process you will transform into being and again feeling as if you are becoming the young man, virile, alive, and filled with energy for life.

You are becoming that man. You love the new the new younger and more alive attitude. This comes from your change in lifestyle, in your change in diet and nutrition. And day by day you see your desired goals coming true.

You see and feel results within you as you are in the process of change. And this process is amazingly automatic, because once you allow me to instruct your subconscious mind through this method, your subconscious mind will automatically begin to make those changes that you desire.

You like the changes, because you are transforming, day by day, into the younger, more vital, more virile person - that person you desire to be.

And as you do so, you relax even more — and as I count down from 10 to 1 you will go deeper. Counting down now,

10- deeper, deeper, deeper, down, down down, deeper, deeper, deeper.

9- totally relaxed, completely relaxed, deep into the deepest levels of mind.

8- deeper, deeper, deeper, down, down, down, deeper, deeper, deeper

7- more and more relaxed, completely and totally relaxed.

6- deeper, deeper, deeper, down, down, down, deeper, deeper, deeper.

5- more and more relaxed …

4- deeper, deeper, deeper, down, down, down, deeper, deeper, deeper.

3 – more and more relaxed,

2- deeper, d-e-e-p-e-r, v-e-r-y d-e-e-e-p now. Down, d-o-w-n, d-o-w-n, deep asleep.

1-and you are deep, deep, asleep.

In your deep level of relaxation now, you have noticed that you've attained your own state of inner peace. From this wonderful state of relaxation and inner peace, you know how to direct yourself to intuitively be involved in the right things at the right time to always get the best results.

Starting this very moment, your confidence, self-esteem, self-worth, all show when people look at you. You can look them in the eye, smile, and then – they see your sparkle, your charm, your charisma and you know that you have the talent and skills to enchant and enamor them. It is your sex appeal and virility that shines through.

And as you go deeper you feel your body working more in harmony with your mind. Because for a while now you had concerns that you were developing Andropause and symptomatically it appeared that way. And although we all know that the declination of Testosterone is a normal thing that the body goes through as you age, it is not necessarily mandatory that you experience this. And, you have gone through the self-evaluation, you have gone through consultation with your physician, and you are on the path to help yourself achieve a natural self-help, using the power of your mind to bring your emotions back in accord, and with them – the chemicals and hormones of your body that had been changing.

Andropause, that you used to struggle with, was a result of a drop in Testosterone – but that's all changing.

Yes, that is all changing through the use of the methods in this book, and with hypnosis therapy because with hypnotherapy and visualization skills you have the power and ability to once again gain control of all your body's emotions, and all of the chemicals in your body.

You will do this because you desire to be healthier, to feel better, and to once again enjoy your life as you have enjoyed it in the past.

Yes, from time to time you might feel some old symptom returning – but by using the hypnotherapy that you are now learning, those symptoms will become less and less frequent, easier for you to manage, and soon, they completely disappear.

Now, allow yourself to go deeper, and d-e-e-p-e-r into those peaceful depths of total and complete relaxation as you listen only to the sound of my voice. My voice guides you, guides you, and leads you, leads you, into the total and complete depths of complete and total relaxation. Deeper and deeper, deeper and deeper.

Sounds around you just fade into the background and have no impact on you whatsoever, you continue to go into the deepest depth of complete and total relaxation, deeper, and deeper, and deeper asleep.

Andropause symptoms vary, but are driven by the same cause – and that you is slowly, day by day, disappearing because the production and release of the hormone Testosterone produced in your testes and regulated by the pituitary gland are now 100% under your conscious control. Right now, see yourself as one. You have total control and their body and mind.

Realize that starting today – you are able to regulate the manufacture and distribution of your own hormones, and you have control over the network of distribution. YOU ARE THE BOSS OF THIS SYSTEM.

Pause (30 seconds)

As you know, your Testosterone is controlled by the different parts of your brain which dictate the process and communicate to your testes how much Testosterone to produce.

This is accomplished through the release of other hormones into the bloodstream that mix together inside your testes and the net result is the production of Testosterone.

Now, I want you to imagine that there is going to be a process by which you can do the repair work yourself, while you are in this relaxed, altered state of mind.

So, now I want you to imagine that you are in special gear, a white wet suit geared up with two tanks on your back. Each of you is carrying a small attached case in colors that match your outfits. Each bag contains all the tools to fix lack of production of Testosterone, flashlight, magnifying glass so you can look closely at the cellular structure – everything that you would ever need to do the repair and test the system.

And with you is a spiritual surgeon who is a specialist in male reproduction. He is in a blue wet suit, and both of you are going to enter your body and locate to the blood stream, in miniaturized form, and you will travel with the red blood cells through your body, by entering your body through your mouth, traveling down the esophagus into the stomach, into the intestines, absorbed through the intestinal walls into the blood stream, through the veins and arteries, and after a long voyage of floating and talking to each other about this therapy – you arrive in the testicles.

(Pause)

And you and this remarkable surgeon are in the testicles to perform maintenance work. You take one testicle and the surgeon takes the other.

The surgeon explained the procedure – and you follow it now. One tank on your back contains a glowing orange fluid which you will spray on all of the cells and vessels of the testicle you are assigned. This orange healing fluid is from the most modern laboratory known to man and science and use of the chemical is restricted only to those who use this audio with the spiritual surgeon.

Now, I want you to watch as the spraying takes place. Watch the surgeon, in his pocket he has one of these small spray nozzles that works with gravity feed and with a pull of the trigger on the nozzle – the orange fluid sprays to cover every single millimeter of the testes, and miraculously starts things working again at the rate of normal production for a man in his 30's. Watch this process taking place. Watch this process successfully taking place. All maintenance necessary is done by the magical orange healing fluid.

Let your subconscious mind work with you and the surgeon, making your system normalized and age regress the system through the use of this miraculous orange fluid that you and the surgeon have sprayed on and watched it miraculously heal all issues and increase the production of Testosterone for you.

Now, go down to the bottom of your testicles, and you are at the scrotal sac and you look around. Check to see if there is a cell cluster that is monopolizing your free floating hormones that you use to combine with cholesterol to produce Testosterone.

Look closely, as you remain relaxed, letting your subconscious and the spiritual surgeon's experience guide you to exactly where you need to be to spray most of this miraculous fluid.

Now, watch the process of the cells and see your hormones and cholesterol binding ... see if anything interferes with it and if so – SPRAY IT – with the orange fluid and watch it normalize now.

Sometimes your liver needs to be addressed by you and the surgeon so that it produces the correct amount of the compound required for the control of your Testosterone levels – so we will go there as well before we leave your body.

Do a good review of the testes now. See if anything else requires reparations. If so, use the orange fluid, spray it and repair it. Now, the spiritual surgeon comes over to the testicle you worked on to verify the quality of your work. And, you go over to the testicle he worked on to inspect it. You both laugh.

You change the nozzle to the other tank. This tank has the most amazing radiant white fluid. It comes from a supernatural source, call it the Universe, God, Jesus, Buddha, Mohammed, or any name you have for a connection to a universal source of life. If you have only yourself and your own inner abilities – that's great – the fluid comes from your own inner mind.

The nozzles are now attached to the radiant white flood tanks. Both you and the spiritual surgeon now spray each testicle. He does one, you do the other. You do the one he did first, and he does the one you did first. You walk to the outside of the scrotal sac and you spray there. And a radiant white light now surrounds your scrotum and your testes and your Testosterone production is now clean and the system works perfectly.

Take a second to thank the team. Thank your spiritual surgeon, thank yourself. And now, I'd like the two of you to go to the prostate, and check around there, and spray with the orange fluid and normalize and heal everything there. If there is any abnormality at the present -- the abnormality will become less and less, smaller and smaller, day by day, until it completely disappears. The orange healing fluid makes sure of that. Now you and the spiritual surgeon spray the radiant white fluid on your prostate, and it glows radiant white and your prostate is now healthy and functioning and appearing as that of a healthy 30 year old male.

And the testicles and the prostate are in super condition, and now it's time to go check out the liver and so you find your way to the liver. And you see that the liver has had an interesting life and needs a general maintenance.

That will be performed by you and your spiritual surgeon – you take one end and he takes another and you begin spraying every millimeter with orange fluid and watching with the magnifying glass how each cell transforms, and look closely – all the cells have smiley faces and if you listen closely – they are humming. They are happy. You and the surgeon meet in the middle. You look around and it's a good job.

You swap the nozzle to the radiant white tank, and you do the area the surgeon has covered with the radiant white fluid and he does yours. And the liver glows. And all is well in your Testosterone production system.

And you and the surgeon catch a ride back through the bloodstream to your tongue, and the both of you walk around back and to the base of your skull to examine and verify the condition of your pituitary gland. Just to assure your best health, the surgeon and you both spray the pituitary and the orange fluid normalizes it, and the radiant white fluid keeps it in perfect shape forever. Healthy forever.

Before leaving your body, the surgeon and you go back to the tongue through some throat to nasal to sinus passages up to the brain. And there you see a neon sign that says – HIGHER CONTROL CENTER. And a stairway reaches up to that doorway.

The two of you take the stairs, step by step, up to the doorway, and with each step you take, you become more relaxed and peaceful. You reach the door, open it, and there are two chairs in the middle of the room. Like gaming chairs with controls in the arms – and the room has computer monitors and dials.

This is the Higher Control Center for your life and your health. And now, the doctor takes over, he sees the screens and evaluates your overall health. There is a setting for optimum health for you and that is with the dials pointing straight up center. The doctor gets up and starts fidgeting with the dials and slowly they go to dead on center. You help and you make all the dials optimized to center. And as the dials are optimized straight up to center – you feel younger and stronger. And now the doctor and you go to the computer screens and systems analysis shows that you are in much better health than before. Your hormone levels are normalized and in balance, your sexual drive which is controlled by your hormones is now functioning better than ever before.

With every day that passes – your body and body chemicals operate more like that of a younger man, a healthier man, the 'you' that you are now becoming.

Both you and the doctor check the Higher Control Center, and everything is perfect. You go down the stairway. And you reach the sinus level and you slide down to the mouth and the doctor follows you down. You both are on your tongue and you hop down, and when your feet hit the floor, you are full-sized male humans and the surgeon is next to you. You remove your wet suits and put them and the tools away.

You shake the surgeon's hand, he gives you a hug in return. Job well done and he is gone.

Pause

Now that everything is working as it should, it's time for you to return to the conscious level – and from now on every time you listen to this audio – you have a feeling of strength, virility, well-being, healthfulness – which will remain with you for the rest of your life.

In a moment I will count to you from 1 to 5, and at the count of five you will open your eyes, feel wide awake and in perfect health.

You have an alternative if it is time for you to go to sleep for the night. If it is time to go to sleep, you can ignore all the wakeup suggestions and go to sleep for the night. This is your choice, to wake up now, or to go deep asleep and after you've had a great sleep you will naturally awake and feel fantastic.

Your choice awake or asleep.

1. Feeling good all over.

2. Feeling the life force in your body.

3. You can awaken or go to sleep at the count of five.

4. Number four, you can awaken or go to sleep on the next number. If you awaken, you'll feel better than ever before in your life. If you go to sleep – you will sleep deeply, peacefully and soundly.

5. Number five, it's your choice – awaken or go deeper and deeper asleep. Number 5.

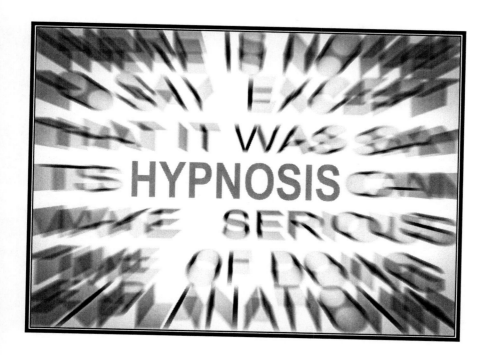

BIBLIOGRAPHY

The Andropause Mystery: Unraveling Truths about the Male Menopause, The Key to Healthy Prostate and Andropause, Robert S. Tan, 2009

How to Cope with Male Menopause -The Andropause Mystery Revealed (HRT - Hormone Replacement Therapy),
Dr. Treat Pearson, 2013

Andropause: What Every Man and Wife Should Know A Guide to Treatment for Male Menopause,
Allan Wagner, 2012

Hard As A Rock,
Dr. Jay Polmar, 2009

http://www.mayoclinic.org/

http://www.wikipedia.com

FOLLOW THE PLAN

1. **Read the book. When finished, read the book again.**

2. Get diagnosed by a qualified healthcare professional(s) if multiple symptoms are evident.

3. **Use only proven Andropause treatments such as the one recommended herein - http://www.provacyl4men.com**

4. Use the Mediterranean diet and/or other suggested natural remedies.

5. **Use vigorous exercise and meditation on a consistent basis.**

6. Use hypnosis for 40 days.

7. **Re-evaluate.**

INDEX

A

Abusing drugs 78
Acceptable Drinks 95
Acceptable Fruit List 94
Acceptable Protein List 95
Acceptable Snacks 95
Acceptable Stimulant List 96
Acceptable Veggie List 94
Adenocarcinoma 72
Adrenocorticotrophin 52
Age-related mid-life crisis 17
Aldosterone 48
Almeida, David 16
Alzheimer 53, 55
Alzheimer's disease 5, 53
Amazon rainforest of Brazil and Peru 79
American Medical Association 115
American stereotype, popular 19
Amounts of Red Meat 90
Androderm 42
Andrology 48-9
Andropausal 25
Andropause 1-31, 33, 35, 37-9, 42, 44, 46-8, 50-52, 54-8, 60, 62, 68-70, 76, 80, 82-126
  developing 118
  experiencing 20, 98
  male 24-5, 64
  mirror 8
  reason 10
  surrounding 46

symptom of   8, 51
Andropause and Erectile Dysfunction   105
Andropause Mystery   126
Andropause phenomenon   7
Andropause Questionnaire   58
Andropause screening   55
Andropause Self-Test   58
Andropause Society   58
Andropause sufferers   27
Andropause symptomology   9-10, 25
Androstenedione   57
Antiglucocorticoid   52
Apples   93
Apricots   93
Asian Journal   48-9
Avena sativa   79
Avoiding Estrogenic   102
Awakening   33

B

B-complex vitamins   83
Bad temper   24
Balance, natural T-level   66
Baltimore Longitudinal Aging Study   53
Baltimore study   53
Bananas   93
Barrett-Connor   49
Beans   94-5
Beet   94
Benign Prostatic   71
Benign Prostatic Hyperplasia see BPH
Bethesda   55
Bibliography   126
BIMC   49
BIMC measures memory   49

Bio-Available Testosterone Starting   8

Bioavailable Testosterone   49-50

Bioavailable Testosterone levels   49

Black Cohosh Root   80

Blueberries   93

BOSS   119

BPH (Benign Prostatic Hyperplasia)   71, 73-4, 80

BPH symptoms   73

Brain Function   31

Brain Involvement   31

Breakthroughs   27

Brisk   97

British Medical Association   115

Broccoli   68

Broiled Seafood   93

Brussels Sprouts   68

Bt11   62

C

Cabbage   68, 94

Calgene   61

California   49

Californian company   61

CaMV   62

Canada   8, 11

Canadian physicians   8

Canadian psychoanalyst   15

Carlson team in Canada   53

Carrot   94

Cauliflower   94

Causations   18

Celery   94

Char-Broiled   90

Chard   94

Chayote   94

Chromosomal examination 41

Cialis 75

Cisgenic 61

Clinic, Cleveland 7

Commercial sales 61

Complex hormonal cycles 24

Congratulations 115

Control Center 123

Cowper's gland 34

Cyclic Guanosine Monophosphate 35

CYP 63

CYP enzyme 64-5

CYP enzyme activity 64

Cytochrome P450 63

D

Daddy 99

Damiana 96

Damiana leaf 80

Decaffeinated Coffee 95

Defining Types Of Erections 32

Dehydroepiandrosterone 1, 48, 52

Dehydroepiandrosterone sulfate 48

Desserts 96

DHEA 48, 52-6

  steroid 53

DHEA and DHEA-S levels 52

DHEA replacement therapy 53

DHEA secretion 53

DHEA supplement therapy 54

DHEA Therapies 54

DHEAS 48, 54

DHT 34-5, 56, 71-3

Diagnosing Andropause 46-7, 49, 51, 53, 55, 57, 59

Diagnosis of BPH 71

DIE Validity of research   26
Diet   82-3, 85, 87-9, 91, 93, 95, 97
Diet, classic Mediterranean style   93
Diet Drinks   95
Dihydrotestosterone   34, 55, 71-2, 80
DIM   68
Dindolymethane   68
Dionysus   90
DNA   60, 62
   damaged   84
   modified   63
DNA microarrays   62
DNA repair   84
Dopamine   32
Dopamine function   32
Dosage   80, 85
Drink Red Wine   89

E

Early Prostate Problems   74
Early Research   13
EFAs (essential fatty acids)   83
Effects of Andropause   5
Eggplant   94
Elevated Estradiol levels   50
Elk Antler Velvet   80
Empty nest syndrome   18
Emulate   91
Epidemiological comparisons   50
Estradiol   49-50, 55, 57
   bioavailable   49
   low   50
Estrogen   10, 12, 34, 43-4, 48-9, 56, 66-8, 72-4, 80, 102
   little   73
   mimic   66

traditional   44
Estrogen hormone   74
Estrogen levels   68, 83
Estrogen replacement, using   48
Estrogen therapies   44
Estrogenic   67
Estrogenic activity   68
Estrogenic compounds, avoiding   102
Estrone   57, 74
  helping metabolize   74
Examine.com   23
Excess Estrogen   71-2
Exercise   82-3, 85, 87, 89, 91, 93, 95-7
Expel Xenohormones   66
Exposed   40

F

FAI   57
Family Affair   103
FDA   42
Feta   89
Fiber Bars   95
Fifty   26
Flavored Soy Milk   95
Flavr Savr   61
Flax   68
Follicle Stimulating Hormone (FSH)   56
France   55
Francisco, San   44
Free Androgen Index   57
FREE-PSA   43
Free Testosterone method   57
Friendships   21
FSH (Follicle Stimulating Hormone)   56

G

Gazpacho   93
Germany   58
Ginkgo   80
Ginkgo Biloba   80
Ginseng   96
GLORY   22
Glycosophate   65
Glycosophate residue   65
Glycosophate use   65
GM animals   61
GM crops   61
GM foods   60-62
GM plants   61-2
GMO events   61
GMOs   61, 63
GMOS Genetic Modification   60-61, 62, 65, 67, 71, 73, 75, 77, 79, 81
Gokhru fruit   80
Gotu cola   80
Grapes   93
Great Britain   27
Greek   93
Greek salad   91, 93
Green Beans   94
Green Chili   94
Green Olives   94
Green Peas   94
GT73   62
Guavas   93

H

Heart-Healthy Fat   91

Heart Risks   12

Heinemann, Lothar   58

Heller, Carl   13

Heraclitus   2

Herbal Tea   95

Heredity   72

Hip fractures   11

Hormonal Normalcy   24

Hormone Estrogen   5

Hormone replacement therapy (HRT)   12, 41, 44, 126

Horney Goat Weed   96

Hot coffee   67

HRT see hormone replacement therapy

Human Development and Family Studies   16

Hyperplasia   71

Hypogonadism   1, 7-8, 39-42, 49, 101

  extreme   7

  male child   46

  male youth   41

  term   9

I

IGF   48

Impact Of Andropause   30, 32, 34, 36

Improving memory   48

Indian Ayurveda practice   23

Indian cultures   17

Inhibited CYP enzymes   64

Interference   33

J

Janowsky   51

Janowsky team   50

Jaques, Elliott   15

Jicamas 93

K

Kale 68
Kalmijn Netherlands 53
KRON 44

L

L-arginine 85
Late-onset Hypogonadism 7-8
LDL cholesterol 88, 90
  removing 89
Lebanese hummus 91
Legendary Austrian neurologist 15
Lemonade 95
Lemons 93
Lentils 94
Lentils works 68
Leydig 1
Leydig cells 1, 34
  receptive 38
LH (Luteinizing Hormone) 1, 37, 56
LIFE Symptoms 9
Lignans 68
Limes 93
Loss of erectile function 76
Loss of short-term memory 25
Low T-levels 27, 41-2, 69
  male 12
Low Testosterone levels 6, 10, 27-9, 41, 102
Lower Testosterone levels 11, 26, 101
Lowered vitamin D3 levels 64
Luteinizing Hormone (LH) 1, 36, 56
Lycopene 84

M

Maca   79
Maca root powder   80
MAGICAL Fresh Fruits   88
Magnesium   83
Male Menopause Buzzes   13
Man   9, 72, 126
Mandarins   93
Manganese   83
Mango   93
MART (menopausal androgen replacement therapy)   44
Maryland   55
Mayo Clinic   26
MED   93
MED program   93
Median age   52
Mediterranean   88, 92
Mediterranean chef   91
Mediterranean coast   86, 89-90
Mediterranean coast grilling   90
Mediterranean diet   85-6, 88-93, 103
Mediterranean lifestyle   92-3
Mediterranean People   91
Mediterranean people love nuts   89
Mediterranean seacoast   89
Mediterranean states   86
Mediterranean style cooking   90
Melons   91, 94
Men   8, 11, 19, 25, 29, 41, 70, 73, 79, 100, 102
Mid-Life Crisis and Andropause   22
Mid-life Crisis and Erectile dysfunction   22
Mid-Life Crisis Study   17
Mid-life Crisis Prevention   21
Mini Mental State Examination   49

Mini Mental Status Examination   53
Mohammed   122
Molehills   98
Mon810   62
Morley   50
Moroccan couscous   91
MS   76
Muira puama   79-80
Myers, Gordon   13

N

Native Americans   80
Nectarines   94
Niacin   80
NIH   55
Nitric oxide   35
   producing   85
North Americans   90-93
Northwestern Memorial Hospital in Chicago   7

O

Ohio   7
OMG   35
Orangeade   95
Oranges   94
Organic Failure   9
Orgasms   36
Overtime   13

P

Panax Ginseng   80
Papayas   94
Parabens Parabens   66

Patches, transdermal Testosterone   50
PCR (polymerase chain reaction)   62-3
PCR assays, real-time   63
Peaches   94
Pears   94
Pearson   126
Penn State   16
Personal expectations   18
Personal indeterminacy   24
Peruvian root   79
Phytoestrogens   68
Plums   94
Polycythemia   43
Pomegranates   68, 94
Portuguese   92
Procrastination   22
Production, intuitive ALPHA/THETA brainwave   109
Progesterone   56, 79
Propylene Glycol and Polyethylene Glycol   67
Propylene Glycol and Polyethylene Glycol Years   67
Provacyl 37-8, 104, 127
Prunes   94
PSA   56
  high   42
PSA exam   42
PSA levels   42, 56
Psychogenic   32

Q

Quality Of Life Symptoms   9
Quoted   60

R

Radish   95

Raisins   94
Rancho Bernardo   49
Recognized/Under Diagnosed   55
Recommended herbs   74
Red Bull   83
Red clover extract   79
Red grapefruit   84
Reduce/Eliminate List   96
Reflexogenic   33
Reflexogenic and Spontaneous erections   33
Renin   48
Rivermead Behavioral Memory Test   53
Rock   126
Rounded Shoulders   11
Roundup   65
Roundup Ready (RR)   62-3
RR (Roundup Ready)   62-3

S

SDG (Secoisolariciresinol Diglycoside)   68
SEAFOOD & FISH   89
Secoisolariciresinol Diglycoside (SDG)   68
Seduce   101
Seeds   93, 95
Sex Hormone-Binding Globulin   8
Sex Life   31
Sexual maturation   39
Sexual stimulation   33
SHBG (sex hormone binding globulin)   8, 37, 42, 64
SHBG, blood protein   37
Sigmund Freud   15
Smoking   78, 81
South America   79
Soybean Curd   95
Spanish Gazpacho   91

Spinach   95
Spontaneous erections   33
SRT   50
SSBG (sex steroid-binding globulin)   37
SSRI antidepressants   35
Starfruit   94
Starbucks loyalist   67
STARTERS   90
Stinging nettle root   79
Strawberries   94
Styrofoam   67
Styrofoam cup   67
Sulfate   66
Sulfates Sodium Lauryl Sulfate and Sodium Laureth   66
Sunderland team   53
Super Dietary Supplement   85
Supplements, Taking DHEA   54
Symptom Research   27
Symptomology Impacts   9
Symptoms of Andropause   46, 51-2, 57-8, 80, 119

T

T-Level, male   26
T-levels   12, 26-7, 39, 42, 51, 57, 66, 79, 82, 96
   bioavailable   50
   high   50
   lower   27
   normal   26
Tan, Robert S.   126
Testicular biopsy   41
Testoderm   42
Testosterone   1, 5-6, 8-9, 23, 26-8, 32-5, 38-40, 42-3, 48-51, 56,
      70-73, 79-80, 84, 96, 118-19
   bio-available   7, 9, 42
   blood   57

circulating 8

converting 102

experiencing lowered 9

free 48-9, 79

help synthesize 84

hormone 119

hormones 1

important 101

little 73

low 28, 35, 57, 101

male 72

misuse 43

natural 79-80

normal 42, 44

production of 1, 36, 120-22

releasing 84

Testosterone declining 101

Testosterone deficiency 7, 58

Testosterone depletion 11

Testosterone gels 27

Testosterone levels 1, 6, 8-9, 26, 29, 36, 41, 44, 46, 57-8, 121

healthy 32

healthy adult male 26

interpreting 58

low free 44

measuring 58

normal 48

reduced 15

total 49-50

Testosterone production system 43, 123

Testosterone-protein binding 79

Testosterone receptors 42

Testosterone Replacement 42, 69

using 42

Testosterone Replacement Therapy 41, 44, 58, 69

Testosterone supplement usage 43

Testosterone Supplementation   69
Testosterone supplementations   70
Testosterone supplements   69
Testosterone synthesis   96
Testosterone therapy   27, 42
   using   55, 69
Testosterone to Estrogen ratio   102
Testosterone works   39, 41, 43, 45
Testosterone's role   11
TIME magazine articles   13
Traditional Chinese   22
Traditional Chinese Herbology   23
Transgenic plants   62
Treatment of Prostate Problems   73
Tribulus Terrestris   23
Triiodothyronine   48
Tuna   83
Turkish Tabouleh   91
TV   92
TV dinners   67

U

United States   7, 24, 27
Universe   113-14, 122
Unraveling Truths   126
US Census Bureau   29
US government   75
Using Testosterone   43, 55

V

Vegetable Juices   95
Verifying Barrett-Connors   50
Viagra   75
Viagra prescription and Viagra   78

Viagra works   85
Vitamin B12   89

W

Wagner, Allan   126
Watercress   95
Western societies   17
White Breads   96
White Flour   96
White Rice   96
Wikipedia   1, 61
Wolf's Team   55
World Health Organization   1, 5, 24, 29

X

Xenobiotics   64
Xenoestrogens   66-8, 102-3
  causing   67
Xenohormone   66

Y

Yanase group in Japan   53
Yoga exercises   97
Yohimbe   96

Z

Zinc   80, 83-4
Zucchini   95

CPSIA information can be obtained at www.ICGtesting.com
Printed in the USA
BVOW04s1713120514

353286BV00017B/596/P